M000211561

CONGRATS DAD!

A Guidebook for Expectant Fathers

MR. ASHIYA

© Copyright 2020 - All rights reserved.

The content contained within this book may not be reproduced, duplicated or transmitted without direct written permission from the author or the publisher.

Under no circumstances will any blame or legal responsibility be held against the publisher, or author, for any damages, reparation, or monetary loss due to the information contained within this book, either directly or indirectly.

Legal Notice:

This book is copyright protected. It is only for personal use. You cannot amend, distribute, sell, use, quote or paraphrase any part, or the content within this book, without the consent of the author or publisher.

Disclaimer Notice:

Please note the information contained within this document is for educational and entertainment purposes only. All effort has been executed to present accurate, up to date, reliable, complete information. No warranties of any kind are declared or implied. Readers acknowledge that the author is not engaged in the rendering of legal, financial, medical or professional advice. The content within this book has been derived from various sources. Please consult a licensed professional before attempting any techniques outlined in this book.

By reading this document, the reader agrees that under no circumstances is the author responsible for any losses, direct or indirect, that are incurred as a result of the use of the information contained within this document, including, but not limited to, errors, omissions, or inaccuracies.

Table of Contents

Introduction

Hello, and let me be one of the first to congratulate you on your new status as an expectant father.

Not that you did much to get this newfound status, or will be doing any of the tougher tasks during the pregnancy. In fact, all you did to get here was have some sex.

That last sentence was not meant to take away any of the joy you should be feeling, but rather one of the strange emotional experiences you might be having at the moment. And I should know, as I've been through this process twice now. That's my main qualification for writing this book, in fact. I'm not a doctor, nor a registered life coach, but just another dad. As such, you can expect many of my own adventures in becoming a father in this book.

I decided to write it because at the time there was nothing like it. Being readers, both my wife and I headed for the nearest bookstore after that pregnancy test came back positive. There was an entire shelf dedicated to her journey, but nothing for me. It was her idea to document my adventure(s) in fatherhood.

For now, back to your role in the pregnancy thus far. I'm downplaying your role, because that's how I felt in the beginning, right after we started telling people. I'd get handshakes, hugs, pats on the back and even presents, but I felt like a fraud. All I did was have sex with my wife, which seemed like an odd thing to be praised for.

To me, that's a common thing for a dad during a pregnancy. After the conception, there's not much for you to do. Your wife is going through the magical experience of creating life, and you're essentially benched for nine months.

That was my thought process during our first pregnancy, and I can tell you right now that it's absolute rubbish. There's no denying the fact that a woman does the brunt of the work when it comes to pregnancy, but you have a significant role to play as well. Both before and after.

Rid your mind of any notion that you're simply nothing more than a sperm factory. You might not feel that important at the start, but let me assure you that you have a lifetime of hard work ahead. At some point you'll be looking back at these initial emotions and laugh at yourself.

Allow me to rather congratulate you on wanting to improve yourself in anticipation of the arrival. The very fact that you chose this book, and want to know more about what it takes to be a dad, makes you more qualified than most. You should be proud of the fact that you're already taking an interest in your child, even though your child is no bigger than a peanut. That's worth a pat on the back. There are far too many fathers who simply have no interest in their children.

The National Fatherhood Initiative's statistics reveal how dire the situation is. According to their annual report, compiled from data received from the U.S Census Bureau, there are 19.7 million kids growing up without a father present. That's more than one out of every four children in the U.S. In other countries around the world, the statistics are even worse.

There are numerous studies proving that life without a father figure can lead to psychological problems later in life. The fact that you are here, present, and ready to learn how to be a dad already makes you a fantastic father in my book. You've already done so much more than just having sex.

For the record, that's the most depressing section of this book. From here on out, you can look forward to positive reinforcement, some first-hand advice, funny anecdotes and self-deprecating humor. That's right, I'm going to make fun of myself at certain points in this book, because I've made some mistakes. You will too.

Before we move forward, I'd like to share some of my favorite baby facts.

Baby Facts

The world record for the number of births from a single woman is 69 children. She was never named, however. Records from the Monastery of Nikolsk names her as a peasant woman from the village of Shaya in Russia. According to these records, she had seven sets of triplets, 16 sets of twins and four quadruplets. The record for the father with the most biological children belongs to Feodor Vissilyev, the above-mentioned peasant woman's husband. After her death, he married another woman and had 18 more kids.

Even though these births are well-recorded, modern scientists aren't convinced that this could have happened, and it's impossible to investigate the lineage, since this supposedly happened in the late 1700s.

I include this fact to give you hope. Yes, a baby is extremely hard work, but whenever it feels overwhelming, think of Vissilyev's poor wife.

Let's move on to more modern times. According to the current figures, 255 babies are born every minute worldwide. On the flipside, only 107 people die every minute worldwide.

On average, children can't remember the first three years of their lives by the time they're fully grown adults. The leading theory on why this happens is that as babies develop the ability to understand language, they start to build memories differently. The previous memories, built from nonverbal interactions, start to fade.

On the topic of memory, babies can remember the time they spent in the womb. New sounds tend to startle them, but they tend to remember the things they heard while growing. That's why a baby often isn't startled by music, a dog barking or voices. For the record, babies find the mom's voice the most soothing.

Babies can also develop self-awareness at a young age. The easiest way to test whether your baby is self-aware is to place a small sticker on their forehead. If they reach for the mirror, they're not quite there yet, but if they touch the sticker on their forehead, they already possess some form of self-awareness.

Now we move on to two extremely interesting facts that will give you some idea of what to expect in the coming months and years.

From the time they're born to the time they're fully potty trained, the average baby will go through around 8,000 diapers. That's around 55 packs of diapers, costing roughly $18 each, which equates to a nice round total of $1,000 over roughly four years.

Babies are born without a biological clock, and studies show that parents lose around six months' worth of sleep during the first two years.

Get Some Sleep

This is my first bit of advice to you, dear reader. Put down this book right now and get some sleep. If you're already in bed reading this before you go to sleep, put it down right now and go to sleep. Do it. The rest of the chapters will still be here when you get back.

It seems strange for an author to urge you to put their book down, but after that baby is born you won't sleep properly again for the rest of your life. You might think it gets better once they're teenagers, at college or living their own lives with their own families, but it doesn't. My own mother is still on my case, even though I'm in my mid-30s. When I'm off somewhere exploring the world, she's not able to settle down for the night unless I send a message saying that I'm safe in my hotel room. Because of different time zones, I've often had to lie to her, but as a parent myself, I do understand what it means to her. Being a parent means worrying for the rest of your life, especially once they're out there in the big world, and you have no control over their actions.

But back to babies. Let me give you a few examples of how you'll be losing sleep in the coming years.

Let's start with newborns. They sleep around eight hours a day and eight hours at night. That's 16 hours out of a 24-hour day. Sounds glorious, doesn't it?

Problem is, those eight hours aren't in one go. A newborn's stomach is extremely small, and a full feeding is only enough to get them through three hours. This is perfectly fine during the day when you're awake, but nights are less fun.

Babies don't have a body clock, but we do. For us it's not a case of chugging some milk and then falling asleep immediately. It's a complete disruption of your sleeping pattern, which means you don't get the same quality sleep you did before.

Add to that your elevated senses. Your brain knows there's a newborn in the house, so it assumes that every sound is the baby waking up for a feeding. More often than not, it's just the dog walking around, the wind, or any of the other numerous things that make noise in the night.

Personally, I never felt as if I was 100% asleep. I was somewhere on the verge of fading away, and listening for any sounds that might indicate that the baby was awake.

Eventually a baby will sleep through the night, but there are no guarantees. My second child started sleeping through at three months and has been an amazing sleeper ever since.

My firstborn was a completely different story. The older they get, the more time they spend awake. And because of that infernal non-existent body clock, those awake hours don't always align with your awake hours.

At around eight months old, my firstborn would wake at 2 a.m., ready to get the day started. We tried every tactic, but he just wouldn't go back to sleep. He wasn't hungry, didn't require a diaper change, or any of the other basic needs of a baby. He simply wanted some company. So there I was, wide awake in the middle of the night keeping my son company. He had a wonderful time, because he could go back to sleep later in the day. I had to go to work.

This lack of sleep has an obvious effect on a relationship. You and your spouse are both sleep-deprived, and there's no real solution to the problem. You could do it in shifts, but I always felt guilty about sleeping while my wife was awake, and she had the same problem.

The result is a never-ending argument about the most insignificant things. It was much better the second time around, mostly because we were psychologically prepared for what was to come.

That's why I include this segment on sleep at the very beginning of this book. Know that sleep will be scarce in the coming years. Make peace with it now, and it will be less of an issue when you get there. Also know that you and your spouse will have arguments over stupid things. It is inevitable. We once had an argument about how the diapers were stacked in the dresser drawer. There was no obvious upside to having them stacked upright or flat, yet we had a massive fight in the early hours of the morning.

Talk about it now, before it inevitably happens. Know that you'll be getting on each other's nerves, and accept that there's no real solution to the problem. Sure, there are some books that advise you to implement conflict resolution in that moment, but I knew my wife too well to try and do that. Trying to get her to meditate and talk about her feelings in the middle of the night would have resulted in me being bludgeoned by the nearest heavy object. In our case that would have been a large pot of baby bum cream.

The best advice I can give is to not hold on to the anger you feel in that moment. Sleep it off, and start new every single day. Recognize that your spouse is going through the same thing you are, and rather than defend your stance on diaper stacking, just let it go.

Sounds hectic, doesn't it?

That's why I need you to get some sleep. Nobody with kids will judge you for saying no to an invite. Trust me on this. If you respond to an invite by saying that you and your spouse are rather going to spend the weekend resting, there won't be any snide remarks. In fact, I think you'll be a hero.

There will be no need to convince the wife to get some extra rest. Studies have shown that the amount of energy needed to grow a baby on a daily basis is equivalent to the amount of energy long-distance runners use on short-distance marathons. Basically, she's going to be tired all the time and you won't need to convince her to spend as much time as possible in bed.

So, get up, go to bed and go to sleep. Chapter 1 will be here waiting in a few hours.

Chapter 1: Sharing the News

When it comes to sharing fantastic news, the standard is to do it as soon as possible. As soon as you got that first job, you phoned your parents. The same is true for a new house, car, dog, cat or even a goldfish. It's the most natural thing in the world to want to share great news with loved ones.

Yet, it's different when it comes to babies. Even though this is your first child, you've probably heard that you should wait a few weeks to tell everyone. The thinking behind this is a bit morbid for my taste.

The average waiting period recommended by various parenting websites is 13 weeks. That's when the risk of miscarriage drastically declines. It means you can then tell your loved ones without fear that you might lose the baby.

To me, this defeats the purpose of having loved ones. I'm not suggesting you post a picture of a positive pregnancy test moments after you peed on it, but you can let your inner circle know. My reason for this is the exact opposite to the above standard recommendation.

Why? Well, it's all about support. Going through a miscarriage after a few weeks takes a huge emotional toll on both parents, and it's only natural to want support during such a difficult time. The rest of the world need never know, but a select few will help you through the dark days.

I'm not talking out of experience. Both my boys were perfectly fine throughout, but I do have a close friend who went through three miscarriages before a perfectly healthy bouncing baby girl was born. After the first miscarriage, they decided to follow the 13-week rule. During the second and third his wife relied heavily on him for support. He had to stay strong, giving her the courage to move forward.

Here's the thing, however. He needed support as well, and luckily he came to me. He told me the story of the three previous failed pregnancies a few days after finding out about number 4. We never talked about it again, but I'm guessing the wait for those initial 13 weeks to pass must have been agonizing. Mostly, we just sat and drank coffee, talking about this and that. Just having someone know that you're hurting already eases the burden.

Those are the positives and negatives of when you should tell people. As you can tell, I'm in favor of telling close loved ones as soon as possible, but waiting for that 13-week threshold to tell the rest.

How to Share the News

We didn't have much choice in the matter. Being the firstborn children in both our families, we were the first to get married. To say there was pressure to produce a grandchild is the understatement of the century. The ink on the wedding registry had barely dried before my mother started asking when she could expect her first grandchild.

Unfortunately for her, she had to wait a bit. We wanted a few years all to ourselves. See the world, and get drunk at quiz night without having to worry about sleeping through an entire Sunday.

On one of our holidays, we decided the time was right. We went home and put the plan to action. Around a month later, my wife noticed some changes in her body, so we did the test, and it was positive. After our first appointment at the gynecologist two days later, we were told she was already six weeks pregnant. In other words, it happened on the vacation when we decided we were finally ready to take the big step toward full-blown adulthood. That's also why I tell most people my firstborn was both planned and not planned.

We decided to share the news with our parents sooner rather than later. My wife really wanted to share the news with her mom, and I had been keeping my own mom waiting for five years.

Our method was pretty simple. We purchased baby shoes, put them in a box and gave each one a box. My wife's mom started crying, my mom gave a shriek of joy, but my father gave them both a confused look, wondering why he just received a shoe that was obviously way too small for him to use. It took a few seconds, but he eventually got there.

There are thousands of examples to be found online. It turned out to be one of my favorite parts of researching this book. If ever you need cheering up, and you're sick of cat videos, Google pregnancy announcement images. There's some amazing stuff out there, and you'll inevitably find some sort of inspiration.

My advice is to share the good news with close family and friends first. Then, when you feel comfortable, you can let the world know via social media.

Be warned, however. Once that announcement is made, the floodgates open and unsolicited advice starts flowing in.

Dealing with Advice

This is a tricky part of the pregnancy to negotiate, because most advice comes from a good place. It's simply other people trying to share their own experiences, and what worked for them. The problem is that it's too much, and most of it is completely outdated.

We found that most of our friends our age who already had kids didn't have much advice to dole out. If I recall correctly, the only useful piece of advice I received was to have a diaper party. I'm not one for new-age gender reveals and such, but he explained the benefits. You have a small get-together at your house for all your male friends on the same day the baby shower for the mom happens. Not only do you get to hang with your mates, but the entrance fee of one bag of diapers for each person should sort you out for a few months.

It's a bit of a sham, and I'm slightly embarrassed to admit it here, but it works like a charm. Remember at the beginning when I told you how much diapers cost? Now toss those ethics out the window and send out invites to a diaper party.

Most of the odd advice came from the older generation. It started with things like, "don't you dare lift anything heavier than a teaspoon." Only one problem with that. My wife is a strong, independent woman. She knows more about power tools than I do. When something needs to be done around the house, she's the one to do it. Telling her that she couldn't use a hammer anymore just wasn't going to cut it.

The rest of the advice is silly superstition, carried over from generation to generation. She was told to avoid any form of excitement, whether it be a movie, book or music. Also, she shouldn't lift her arms above her head. Apparently the former leads to birth defects, while the latter tangles the baby up in her intestines.

Other pieces of advice include no hot drinks, because it will boil the baby. The tip that you should eat for two is also a myth. Just think about it from a basic biological perspective. At most, the average woman needs no more than 2,400 calories per day. A growing baby needs around 300.

The above advice is easy to ignore. You simply nod your head, say thank you for the tip and laugh about it later when you're alone. But some pieces of advice are way too personal and intrusive. Some pieces of advice even cause damage over time.

There were a few moments when people got close to the line, but there are three examples of advice that definitely went too far. This advice didn't just cross the line, it took a five-pound sledgehammer to it.

The first was advice on how to induce labor. This piece of advice haunts me to this day, because it feels as if it came from a cartoon, rather than any sort of scientific source. Basically, this person told my wife to sniff pepper if she felt the baby was taking too long to come out. This would induce a sneezing fit, which would put pressure on the lower part of her body and the baby would simply pop out. Another one of those smile and nod moments.

The moment the line was obliterated was when my wife's vagina became the subject of a discussion during the baby tea. I wasn't present, but I can only imagine how awkward it must be once your private parts are discussed the same way normal people would comment on the weather.

First, my wife was told to go for a full Hollywood wax. The reason being that the baby could get carpet burn on the way out. Secondly, she was urged not to allow me into the room at all. "Once a man sees a baby come out of your hoo hoo, he'll never want to put his penis in there again," I believe was the phrase. I can categorically state that the latter piece of advice is absolute rubbish, and my second child is living proof of that.

In addition to all of this, you have to understand that there's an extreme amount of pressure on a woman to do things a very specific way.

A pregnancy tends to dominate every social conversation, and often people will make remarks that aren't meant to hurt, but do. Over the course of eight months, we listened to various remarks like, "you don't fully understand motherhood unless you give birth the normal way," or "anybody who doesn't breastfeed should be arrested for child abuse."

As luck would have it, we did both those things wrong. There were complications during the birth of my first son, and even though my wife wanted to give birth naturally, it was not to be. She was out of it, which made me the medical proxy. I was told that if I didn't make the call, I could lose one or both, so it took me no more than a split second to tell them to cut her open. For the record, I saw my wife's intestines, and I still think she's gorgeous.

The other big problem we had was breast feeding. My wife suffered through six weeks of almost no sleep, a constantly crying baby, and mild depression because she felt she was doing something wrong. After a visit to the doctor's office, he told her she wasn't producing enough milk. We had to switch over to formula, which was a giant knock to my wife's ego.

As a dad, my role in this scenario was providing support. I convinced her that these two setbacks were insignificant compared to a lifetime of motherhood. Having said that, I wished I had participated more during pregnancy discussions. Whenever I hear people comment on how vaginal delivery is the only way to real motherhood, and how breast milk should be the only option, I share our story. This stigma of what real motherhood is needs to disappear.

The best advice I can give in addition to the above is to manage expectations. It's good to have a birth plan, but you need to know from the start that there's a very good chance that the plan won't play out like you imagined it would.

It's much better to focus on the end goal. You're not going in there to demonstrate a perfectly planned birth. The goal is to go get your child, and as long as both mother and child come through on the other side happy and healthy, that's all that really matters.

The Calm After the Storm

After telling the family, receiving congratulations, and basking in the glow of the good news, life just returns to normal.

The first part of the pregnancy was strange to me. As a dad, you're not actively involved in the process, and there's not much to do. The nesting phase is still a few months away, your wife can still pretty much do everything she did before, so life continues on as normal.

I settled back into my normal routine of traveling and writing, often forgetting that we had a baby on the way. I desperately wanted to participate, but there was nothing for me to do.

Luckily, I learned from my mistakes. It may feel like you have nothing to do at this point, but you can already prepare for the coming months.

I don't know how things work in your house, but in mine we're all about equality. I have my chores and my wife has hers. One of her weekly tasks is washing clothes, which, I'm ashamed to admit, I knew nothing about.

So when she eventually reached a point where she was too tired to do it, I had no idea how to even operate a washing machine. I mean, what's the difference between a "normal wash" and a "super wash?" Can a wash even be described as super?

I advise you to learn from your wife as early on in the pregnancy as possible. I did this with our second child, and the amount of stress relief was remarkable. Ask her to walk you through her daily routine at home, and see where you can help out.

She's going to be under immense pressure from the third trimester until the baby is at least one year old.

These little bits and pieces you do add up to a huge relief, and it makes you part of the process. It's a win-win for both of you.

Chapter 2: Becoming Responsible

Part of being a great dad is accepting the fact that you have to take care of yourself. I've read too many stories of children losing their dads at a young age, and I'll admit right here and now that it's my biggest fear by far.

Now that I have two kids, I can't imagine not being around to see them grow up, find partners and perhaps have their own children.

Eventually getting there means you have to make responsible choices, which is something I struggled with at first.

To explain why, I first need to tell you a bit about myself. In my previous life, I was an adventure/motoring writer. It was quite a life, but I inevitably put myself in harm's way more often than I probably should have.

I was perfectly content when it was just me and my wife. She knew what she signed up for, and we had a perfect don't ask don't tell policy. As long as I came back in one piece, all was good.

When the kids came along, I started telling myself all sorts of lies in order to believe that I was still being a responsible adult.

And, if all else failed, at least my kids would have a good story to tell their friends about why they didn't have a father. It sounded romantic in my head at the time, but writing it now I realize how stupid it sounds.

My Many Stupid Adventures

Shortly after I found out my wife was expecting, I was off on a work trip to Bangkok. I wanted to cancel the trip, but the tickets were already paid for and my wife wanted life to return to normal as soon as possible. So, off I went.

I don't remember the specifics of the trip, other than I was there to test how a brand-new tire coped on various surfaces. The manufacturer who set up the trip had a whole facility built for this purpose, and they let me loose on it.

I soon discovered that the car I was driving was not equipped with ABS. In case you don't know car lingo, it's basically a system that keeps the brakes from locking up under hard braking. It's probably the most important safety feature on a modern car, since you have zero control over a car with locked wheels. If you know what you're doing, it's also an easy way to induce a skid, which is utterly meaningless, but extremely fun. It was a good day in the office.

The next day we had nothing scheduled, so a few of my colleagues and I decided to see if we couldn't find some of Bangkok's more infamous shops, specializing in pristine knockoffs. I had no interest in a Rolex, but I'm curious by nature so I tagged along. What's the worst that could possibly happen?

After some snooping around, we eventually found the right person. He took us into an unassuming handbag shop with a secret door. On the other side of this secret door was a room full of knockoff watches, and a man with a very large gun.

One of my colleagues opened one of the glass cases to get a closer look, which upset the man with a gun very much. After pointing the gun our way, the manager of the dodgy store intervened and gave us a stern warning.

My death was supposed to be an epic story. Being gunned down in the back of a handbag shop in Bangkok wasn't exactly what I had in mind.

Still, this wasn't a turning point for me.

Around one year later a friend and I got lost while driving on what we thought was a 4x4 trail. As it turns out, it was a footpath. Our journey went on way into the night, and at one point I had to drive my car across a river. Since it was freezing, there was no way to see how deep it was, so I drove across that river blind. The water started seeping in through the door seals, but the car made it through to the other side.

Still, not a turning point.

Freezing water seems to be my kryptonite, because it brought me right to death's door.

I was part of a team doing a documentary on the Sardine Run in South Africa. We tracked the sardines along the shoreline for a few days, but due to the weather being extremely bad, we couldn't dive.

On the third day we went out on a boat in extremely cold weather. The water temperature was down to single digits, and a storm was blowing in. After around 20 minutes of diving, I surfaced. By then the storm was there in full force. Epic winds, rain, lightning and thunder. After bobbing around for a few minutes the boat found me, but we were still missing a few members of the crew.

At this point I was desperate for a pee. As a general rule, you never go in your wetsuit, because you can never get that smell out. So I removed the top half of my suit, did my business and put it back on. It was just long enough for the suit to cool down completely, which meant it was no longer offering protection against the elements.

Hypothermia is a strange thing. You don't feel it at all. Your body just shuts down piece by piece, trying to keep the core warm. I could not work out why the medics were piling blankets on me, while everyone else was shivering. Only once I recovered did I remember that you should start worrying when you stop shivering.

The medic found the closest hotel room to the dock, burst into the room and scared the living daylights out of a friendly Canadian man. After giving him a quick explanation, he was more than happy to stand aside while I was being forced underneath the shower.

That was the closest call of my life so far, but still not enough for that switch in my brain to go off.

I could name at least a handful of examples of incidents that should have made me rethink my attitude towards my own safety, but it took the death of my own dad to get me there.

He never drank, smoked, but hated the idea of exercise. According to him, both jogging and cycling became irrelevant the moment the car was invented. Throw in a love of fatty foods, and a love of all things chocolate-covered and you have the perfect recipe for a massive heart attack.

A heart attack killed him at 53. Apart from the natural grief of losing a father, I couldn't help but put myself in his shoes. If I died at the same age as he did, my one son would still be in high school, the other most likely at college. I don't know about you, but I feel like I still needed my dad at that age. Heck, my life is pretty much stable, and I still feel like I need some fatherly advice sometimes.

As a dad you have a responsibility to look after yourself, because you will be needed in the future. I'm not saying that I don't still do the odd thing for a thrill, but I do it within boundaries. More importantly, I look after myself. I go for an annual checkup at the doctor, and I follow the basic recommendations for living a healthy life.

Acting Responsible

To me, acting responsible comes in many forms.

It can be something as basic as thinking twice before spending money. There are loads of amazing gadgets out there that I desperately want, but never buy.

I'll often visit a gadget shop, end up staring at a pair of cordless noise-canceling headphones for a few minutes, only to walk out again. I wish my current pair of headphones would just break already, so I at least have an excuse to buy a new set.

I constantly worry about spending money, because it played a big role in our decision to have kids. I didn't want to have kids until we were financially stable enough to be able to cater to their every need.

You make a lot of sacrifices being a dad, but allow me to let you in on a little secret. There are at least three days of the year where you get a gift, so don't be afraid to drop some hints. You can take the subtle approach and mention that your headphones are looking a bit tired, or you can take a direct approach and send an Amazon link to the item directly to your wife's phone.

In all seriousness, being responsible is not that hard.

In fact, I see no reason why you shouldn't treat yourself, but only if you're financially secure enough.

The most responsible thing you can do for your kids is to set a good example.

Have a strong work ethic, help out those in need, and treat everyone around you with kindness. Kids learn by example, which should always be at the back of your mind.

Your relationship with your spouse will be the most important example you set.

Being the father of two boys makes this approach especially relevant. I treat my wife as my equal, not just because I believe she is, but in the hope that my sons treat their partners the same one day. The same goes for a daughter. Having a decent father figure, who treats her mother the way she deserves to be treated, will set a standard for future guys who might be interested.

How to be More Responsible

This is more about life in general, rather than being responsible with regards to parenting.

The fact is, many babies are unplanned, but not necessarily unwelcome. It's the perfect excuse to get your affairs in order, man up and become responsible. This is how to be an adult, or at least my own version of adulting.

The first step is taking ownership of your life. Part of life is struggling and failing. An immature, irresponsible person blames everyone and everything but themself, and that needs to change.

Parenting will be the biggest responsibility you will ever face, and once the initial excitement is gone, it's just you, your spouse and the baby. There's no excuse to hide behind, so best make peace with the fact that you can't blame others for your own mistakes now.

My second tip is to spend less time on social media, for various reasons.

Social media is not just a timesuck and the ultimate procrastination tool, but it also tricks your mind into believing that you're not good enough. The moment you start looking at baby things online, social media websites will start feeding you baby-related content. Not all of it is good for you. Some content might be useful, but other articles will highlight all the things that could go wrong. And while you should be aware of the dangers, it's psychologically damaging to be constantly reminded of the dangers.

I had this problem during the first pregnancy, but we'll get to it in a few chapters.

You might want to ask yourself whether there is room for improvement in your professional life. Many people get stuck at a certain level. It might be the joy of being content with where you are, or fear that you might not be able to do a job further up on the professional ladder. Whatever it may be, ask yourself what it is that's holding you back, and whether you can't do something about it. Set some goals and chase them. A promotion will lead to a better financial position, which obviously has benefits for the whole family.

While on the topic of finances, it's worth exploring a budget. It's difficult to calculate the monthly cost of a baby, because there are too many variables to consider. A good ballpark figure is somewhere between $150 to $300 per month. That's excluding the cost of having the baby, and buying all the necessary furniture and gadgets you'll need.

If you can easily absorb that cost, good for you. For the rest, I suggest drawing up a list of expenditures. The list should include both expenditures that you absolutely have to pay, and those that aren't absolute necessities. This will give you a clear indication of where you can cut costs in order to afford the things the baby needs.

And, for goodness sakes, don't buy stuff just to impress on your social media platform. A $125 stroller does the exact same job as a $3,000 stroller.

Chapter 3: Doctors

As a man you've always been aware that gynecologists exist. You might not know the specifics, but you do know that women go to them for "lady problems."

To be perfectly blunt, men don't know much about vaginas at all. I was most certainly guilty of this. Up until my wife's pregnancy, I knew just enough about vaginas to keep myself out of trouble.

Having a pregnant wife means getting a crash course on the intricacies of having a vagina. Man, it's hard work. Every time I left that office, I said a small prayer thanking the higher power for my penis. Not only is it much easier to maintain, but the whole world is your toilet.

That first visit to the gynecologist's office is extremely intimidating, for various reasons.

First and foremost, it feels as if you're treading on sacred ground. As if you're on the 11th floor of a building, but you only have level 6 clearance. And that's just the reception area.

The actual room where the inspections are done is a lot more intimidating. There are graphic posters on the wall, tools you don't understand, and a bed that has these strange extensions for a woman's legs.

The tools bothered me the most. There a large variety of strange objects that would not have looked out of place in a torture scene in a movie. I tried figuring out what each one did, but my overactive imagination sent shivers down my spine.

Luckily, offices like these are equipped for first-time fathers. The doctor pointed towards a little stool next to the bed and told me to sit there. From there I could see the sonar images, chat to my wife, and the doctor, but nothing at the business end. I'm fairly certain gynecologists are aware of how nervous first-time fathers are, and thankful that they ease you into the whole process.

As men we're not accustomed to doctors getting up close and personal with our privates, but it's something women have to deal with from a young age. My wife knew her doctor, so while she was busy going about her business down there, the two of them chatted about the weather, life in general, and where we were going on holiday that year. I was astonished at how casual the whole operation was.

I know my GP well. We're old friends and he's treated me for many ailments over the years, but never something penile related. I'd like to think that if that time finally came, we'd be silent during the whole process and we'd never mention it again.

How to Behave at the Gynecologist's Office

Vagina doctors are very good at spotting first timers.

Apart from the obvious nervous behavior, and the awkward glances at the model's female genitalia, they know you're most likely uncomfortable. You're most definitely not the first man with a pregnant wife, which means they can spot a nervous man from a mile away.

In addition to this, we men have this whole annoying masculinity thing going on. I don't know about you, but my wife has to make me go to the doctor when I'm sick. I'm always 100% convinced that whatever sickness it is, I can simply ride it out. Then it just gets worse, until I eventually give in and end up going a week later than I should have. And I know I'm not the only one who does this.

So why do we do it, guys? I'll go first and be brutally honest. I don't like going to the doctor, because it feels defeatist. I want to prove that my body is stronger than whatever sickness. I'm fully aware that it's idiotic, especially now that we've lived through an actual pandemic, but that's one of the reasons I don't like going to the doctor.

The second reason I don't like going is the expectation of bad news. After my dad's heart attack, his doctors urged me and my brother to go for a round of tests. My grandfather died of a heart attack as well, so the chances of it being a genetic problem were quite high. My brother went immediately, but I put it off for months. I was sure that the news would be bad, and that it would be real the moment I took that test.

This brings us back to being responsible. I had two choices. I could go through life not knowing whether I had the same heart condition, hoping that it wouldn't kill me. Or I could do the test and if the results came back positive, the doctors could do something about it. Wanting to spend as much time with my kids as possible, I went for the second option, and I'm happy to report that my heart is perfectly fine.

All of this only happened after the birth of my second son, so I was still very much a skeptic of doctors when we started going to the gynecologist. Every time she frowned at the screen during the sonar, I was expecting the worst.

And every time it was just something routine. "I'm just trying to get him to move so we can get a better view of his hands," or something along those lines.

The best piece of advice I can give you is to not project your own fears. You're not the center of attention in that moment, and you won't be for a while. Trust in the doctor. He/she has most likely spent decades studying the vagina, while you are nothing more than a fan.

Having said that, don't be afraid to ask questions. The gynecologist will likely respect you more, because you're taking an active interest in the baby and your wife's health. They'll happily talk you through a procedure, or explain the various parts that make up the parts of the female anatomy. This information won't just be helpful during the pregnancy, but also if your baby turns out to be a girl.

A general understanding of private parts goes both ways as well. My wife, being the proud owner of a vagina, had no idea how a penis worked. Other than the basics, obviously.

This became apparent once we started potty training. I came home one day, and she had a whole list of questions about how men urinate. "Do you hold it with both hands?" I nearly died laughing, but then I realized she had no way of knowing. It's not like she needed to know the answer to that question before.

My wife requested the final piece of advice in this particular section. According to her, and all of her friends, women hate it when you refer to 'we' during an appointment. "We're having some problems with morning sickness," or "we're experiencing an elevated sense of smell."

I'm reliably informed that a pregnancy is a singular process. Sure, you can lend a helping hand here and there, but when it comes to incessant vomiting, cramps and cravings, it's just her.

Tips to Help You Help the Mom

In order to be helpful during the initial phase of the pregnancy, you need to understand what your wife is going through. As I explained above, there's still a lot of confusion on both sides, and you can help remedy that by being informed.

The first tip is fairly obvious. Simply attend as many doctor's appointments as you possibly can. The gynecologist is the best source of information, as he/she will talk you through the entire development stage, and explain your baby's growth chart. He/she is the best source of information you have at your disposal, and will answer any questions you might have better than Google.

Any decent gynecologist will recommend a series of lifestyle changes. Some of it will be obvious, like no drinking alcohol, smoking or skydiving. Other changes will be less obvious, like getting exercise, taking additional vitamins, and eating healthier. These rules don't apply to you, but you can implement them in solidarity with your wife. Like I said before, part of being responsible is being present, and healthier habits is the first step toward that goal.

I also strongly suggest joining a weekly pregnancy newsletter, especially if you can't make it to all the doctor's appointments. These weekly newsletters tell you everything you need to know about your baby and your wife on any given week. It's sort of like a cheat sheet for dads who want to help. The newsletter might tell you that your wife may be at the point in the pregnancy where she'll start experiencing lower back pain. Being the thoughtful dad that you are, you can then buy the necessary remedy without even being asked.

Finally, invest in some baby classes. I'm such a big fan of these classes that I decided to dedicate an entire chapter to it.

Chapter 4: Baby Classes

Is it worth investing in baby classes? My answer is undoubtedly yes. Having said that, it took some persuasion to get me there.

Within the first month of finding out I was going to be a dad, I worked my way through *What to Expect when you're Expecting* in both book and movie format. In my mind, I was already an expert.

My wife wanted us to attend just to be sure, and I'm glad we did. There are so many things you learn at these classes that you simply can't learn from a book. Some things are just better suited to a live demonstration, but it goes beyond that.

Soothing Anxiety

Baby classes aren't just about the practical side of raising a baby. They exist to ease the mother and father into the idea of parenthood by demonstrating that raising a child isn't that hard.

The other part that resonated with me was the camaraderie. We attended our classes with 24 other couples, most of whom were also first-time parents. Just knowing we weren't the only people going through this process already helped lower the stress levels.

The first step in the process was to stand up and introduce yourself to the class. You had to say who you were, what you did for a living, and when your baby was due.

I found the variety of jobs the most interesting part of this exercise. There were lawyers, accountants, actuaries, business owners, and even a pharmacist. These are all considered prestigious jobs, mostly done by people who are extremely smart. The fact that they also needed help made me feel less inadequate.

It's also comforting meeting a bunch of people who are going through the exact same thing you are. After every class the various attendees would hover around and drink the complimentary coffee. During this time, we'd share stories of the ridiculous advice received, overbearing grandparents, and where to find the necessary furniture at the best prices.

Best of all was the belief that there were no stupid questions, especially from the dads. Eventually everyone started asking all the questions we were all wondering about, but were too embarrassed to talk about. Like when was it okay to have sex again after the baby is born, and won't I be poking the baby in the head if we have sex during the pregnancy?

Everyone laughed at these questions, but deep down we all were wondering the same things.

And just because I brought it up now, and you've probably wondered about it, the answer is no. You won't be poking the baby in the face when you have sex during the pregnancy.

Below is a list of the information I found particularly useful during baby class.

The Layout of the Hospital

By the time you go for baby classes, you should already have made a decision about where the baby will be born. The vast majority of hospitals offer these classes, and they give you a thorough tour of the facilities, as well as the rules.

This put my mind at ease, because getting my wife to where she needed to go to have the baby was one of the few jobs I had, and I was planning on doing it well. I even went as far as scouting various routes from our house to the hospital, which led to two possible routes depending on what time of the day it was.

The nurse in charge of the class walked us through the whole process, from the moment you drive through the hospital gates. It was a step-by-step process, and she physically walked us through the whole thing.

Simply knowing exactly what you need to do on the big day removes a large chunk of the anxiety. This knowledge alone made the whole thing worth it.

Taking Care of Mom

As mentioned earlier, some lifestyle changes are necessary. These classes covered the basics of good nutrition, as well as the exercises the mother could do during the various stages of the pregnancy.

This segment covered the best sleeping positions, products recommended by doctors, and what you as the father could do to ease the burden.

It also covers the various hormones that will be released into your wife's system, unleashing the hormone monster. More on this in an upcoming chapter.

Early Development and Complications

This covered the trimesters, as well as all the big moments you can look forward to, like the first time the mother will be able to feel the baby move.

It also covers some complications, and the solutions. Luckily hospitals are much better equipped to handle difficult births than they were just two decades ago, so the idea is not to instill any sort of fear. The idea is simply to tell you what can happen, and why it shouldn't cause you any panic if it does.

Sex

There's more to sex and pregnancy than simply knowing when it's okay to get back to it after the baby is born.

Most couples tend to be completely out of sync during the pregnancy. When you're in the mood early on in the pregnancy, she probably won't feel up to it. Later on in the pregnancy she'll be the one who wants to jump your bones, but the belly makes it difficult. I'm not referring to the positions, though they do cover that as well, but rather the psychology of having another person (the baby) in the room.

The thought of bumping the baby with my penis never crossed my mind. My imagination was far more extreme than that. I felt as if the baby was judging us every time we had sex. I could just imagine it thinking what sort of sex-crazed family it was being born into.

Labor and Delivery

As it turns out, this class would be the most important one I would attend.

The nurse walked us through the signs that a woman is going into labor. It's worth paying attention to this particular segment, because many women turn up at the hospital ready to have a baby, only to be sent home because it was a false alarm.

The closer you get to the due date, the more contractions there will be. These are called Braxton Hicks contractions, which basically exist to get the body ready for the delivery.

On paper it's easy to tell the difference between a Braxton Hicks contraction and the real deal, but in real life it's anything but. Braxton Hicks contractions are sporadic, while real contractions happen at regular intervals. A real contraction's pain also starts in a different place than Braxton Hicks.

With that in mind, it should be easy to identify, but keep in mind the stress involved in the situation. Luckily, I was fast asleep on the day it happened.

My wife woke up early, made sure it wasn't a false alarm, and then had a shower. She was calmer than a chicken in a vegan restaurant. She also knew me well enough to know that I would freak out once she told me, which is exactly what I did.

I got her in the car, got us to the hospital in record time, followed all the steps, and eventually we ended up in a delivery room. This was just after 10 a.m. in the morning. As it eventually turned out, my son was still more than seven hours away.

Every once in a while a nurse would come in to check the dilation. We waited for hours, until the doctor eventually decided to manually break her water to induce labor. At this point in time, my wife's heart was still set on a natural birth.

From there things went sideways, but luckily my training from the baby classes kicked in. During class we did a thorough rundown of the possible delivery problems, as well as the solutions.

My wife's blood pressure was extremely slow and my son wasn't moving. Since she was in no shape to make medical decisions, I had to make the call and an emergency C-Section was booked.

I knew where to go, where to sit, and what to do directly after the birth. From the moment I gave the go-ahead to the moment I saw my son for the first time was no more than 15 minutes. It would have been much worse had I not been prepared ahead of time.

For the record, you do watch videos of the birthing process in class. I was scared that I might never want to look at a vagina ever again, but it really wasn't that bad. To look at, I mean. I have no doubt that it's likely the most painful thing a person can do. To put it in perspective, the nurse told us that it was the equivalent of squeezing an orange through your penis.

Before seeing a natural birth, I was always a big fan of the unsolvable pain puzzle. If you haven't heard of it, it's basically a comparison in pain. Is it more painful to give birth, or to get kicked in the testicles? It's unsolvable, because you can never do both. I know which side I'm on, however. I'd much rather take a swift kick in the sack than give birth. It's not even a close competition.

After the Delivery

Some see a C-Section as the easy way out, but the recovery is long, rough and painful.

Thanks to the classes, I knew that I was going to have to take charge for the first few hours while my wife was in recovery. I had no problem with that. When I have a problem, I'd rather face it as soon as possible, which is why I wanted to be the one to change that first infamous diaper. I nailed it, and every diaper since.

I think the expectation of a diaper change is much worse than it is. It also helps that it's your own flesh and blood, making it much easier to cope with the gross factor.

In addition to diaper and clothing changes, I also had to help my wife.

The C-Section may seem like an easier option while giving birth, but the recovery period is so much longer.

My wife shared a room with a woman who gave birth naturally, and by the next day she was able to get out of bed, walk around, and go to the bathroom by herself. With a C-Section, it's a two-person job just to get someone upright. The hospital sent a physiotherapist over to demonstrate the right way to get up, and out of bed. Even when you implement these methods, it still hurts a lot.

Our hospital stay was also lengthened by two days. For a natural birth, a woman tends to spend two days in the hospital if there aren't any complications. The hospital is happy to let you go as soon as you can do a number two.

My wife ended up spending four days in the hospital, before she could work up the courage to go to the bathroom for that very reason. It would have been extremely awkward explaining to the family why we weren't on our way home yet, but I didn't want to put extra pressure on my wife. Imagine having an entire family rooting for you to have a poop.

The recovery at home also takes another six weeks, so be ready to pitch in whenever you can.

Bathing the Baby

The day after the birth, a kind nurse came over to ask if they could use our child for the baby class demonstration on how to wash a newborn. Since we were part of the audience a few months ago, we said yes.

When the time came, I took my son over for his first bath. The nurse who gave the demonstration wasn't the same kind nurse from the morning. I got the sense that she was at the end of her shift, and wasn't really in the mood to demonstrate proper bathing techniques to a bunch of enthusiastic expecting parents.

The whole episode was extremely traumatic, viewed from the other side. My son was crying, and I felt this primal urge to tackle the nurse and take him away.

If you were wondering when that paternal instinct kicks in, it's immediate. From the moment I first held my son, I knew that I'd take a bullet for him.

Going Home

Back when I was a young man I had some money saved up for my first car. As an enthusiast of all things motoring, my priority list for my first car was quite short. In fact, it had only one requirement: what's the most amount of power I could get for the amount of money I had?

I eventually rolled that car on a gravel road on the way to my girlfriend's house. In my mind I was an amazing driver, right up until the moment I lost control of the thing. That's when you reach into your bag of talent and realize that it's not as full as you thought. To be honest, my bag was empty.

That should have been a life lesson, but my first car's successors were even more powerful. After going to numerous advanced driving courses both local and abroad, I eventually learned how to tame these beasts.

The arrival of my son coincided with the arrival of my new company car. Normally I'd opt for something stupidly powerful with a decent infotainment system, but this time I scoured the internet to find the safest car within my budget. It turned out to be a Subaru XV, which was a dreary thing to drive, but it scored top marks in standardized international safety tests.

On that very first drive my wife was mocking me. "Going a little slow, aren't we?" She knew full well that I was a fast driver. Not irresponsible, mind you, just fast.

To me it was physically impossible to overtake, even though I knew the road well, and there was nothing coming the other way. There was just too much on the line. Funny how quickly your mindset changes. Before my son was born, I saw speed signs as mere suggestions. After his birth, I could not bring myself to go over the limit.

These days, when I'm alone in the car, I still like to play at times. Nothing irresponsible, or dangerous to other road users, mind you. Having said that, there's nothing wrong with getting some sideways action when you exit a deserted roundabout.

When my sons are in the car, however, I turn into a sterling example of a law-abiding citizen. I frown at drivers who come speeding past above the limit, even though I know full well that I would be doing the same had I been alone in the car.

What to do When You Get Home

Arriving home, we put our son down on the floor in his Moses Basket.

We had spent eight weeks in baby class preparing for this very moment, so we looked at each other, and uttered the same sentence at the same time.

"What the hell do we do now."

My point is this: baby classes are definitely worth investing in, if only to know exactly what you'll be going through at the hospital.

But nothing can prepare you for the moment you first arrive at home. There aren't any nurses around to help, and the teacher isn't there to tell you what to do.

At that moment you realize that it's now up to you to raise this child, and in order to do so you need to take that first step.

Since my son was fast asleep, I got up and made some coffee. The following steps would not be as easy...

Chapter 5: Bonding With the Baby

As I said before, I often forgot about the pregnancy early on. Since I wasn't carrying it, coping with morning sickness or any cravings, I had no daily reminder that a baby was on the way.

During the first and second trimester, there's not much for dad to do. Being the independent woman she is, my wife kept on driving herself, doing her own chores and picking up loads of things heavier than a teaspoon. It was basically life as usual.

Since I'm a big fan of honesty, I told my wife that I was feeling left out. All the attention was on her and the baby, and rightfully so. I didn't want to take that away from her, but I also wanted her to know how I felt.

Being the wise one in our relationship, she told me to write about it. What eventually started as a series of letters, ended up as a 30,000-word book that will only ever be printed twice. One copy for each of my sons.

Writing helped me bond with my unborn child, because I was imagining him as an older man with whom I could have conversations. Knowing the potential of that little fetus helped me bond on a deep level.

Having said that, it's not the only method I used.

Tips for Bonding With an Unborn Baby

Since I couldn't carry the baby around with me like my wife could, I decided to carry one of the photos from the ultrasound with me. I even took it a step further and transferred the videos from the ultrasound over to my phone. That way I could at least get a small portion of the adoration my wife was receiving.

The photo also served as a nice reminder. Every time I opened my wallet, there was an image of the little blob. I wasn't entirely sure which part of the image was my son, but it's the thought that counted. I highly recommend you do the same.

There are also loads of tips on the internet, and I tried most of them. Some of them worked, others didn't, but I include all of them here. Perhaps you'll find the perfect method that's best suited to your personality and talents.

Talk To The Baby

This is the most common piece of advice out there. Spend some time talking to the belly, so the baby gets to know your voice.

I found this extremely odd, however. I mean, what do you say to a baby? In your 30s you're mostly in a state of existential crisis, and it's not like the baby wants to hear about how confusing and cruel the world can be.

I also tried reading to my wife's belly, but this didn't work either. I despise reading out loud, as I can do it much quicker in my head. Vocalizing the words completely messes with the process, so I end up mumbling the words.

This tactic just wasn't working for me, so I decided talking to my wife was enough for the baby to be familiar with my voice by the time it's born.

Having said that, this might work magic for you, so give it a bash.

Buy Something Unique

As a dad, you're probably imagining your baby a little older. The science shows that us dads do that, because we look forward to the point where we can actively play and engage with the child.

I bought a small BMX, knowing full well that my son would only be able to start using it properly at around five years old. At first glance it makes no sense, but having that BMX around always made me smile. I knew at some point I was going to have a little version of myself that was going to need help learning how to ride a bicycle.

I also bought some unique onesies from wherever my travels took me. In my mind, it was something that was special between the two of us. The chances of someone else gifting a onesie from the Hard Rock Cafe in Barcelona were slim.

Keep Up To Date

As I mentioned earlier, it's worth subscribing to some form of weekly newsletter. It's a wonderful life hack, not just for learning more about your baby, but also your wife's experience during the pregnancy.

I loved the part of the newsletters where they told you what your baby is now capable of. Week by week, it was growing into a real little person, which made it so much more relatable.

Help With The Nesting

Nesting will be fully covered in an upcoming chapter, but for now we can talk about the basics.

After we were married, my wife moved into my house. It was a sad little place, so obviously decorated by a man with zero sense of style. Everything in there served a purpose. Scatter cushions were banned.

I had no problem with my wife redecorating the place. It was her place now as well, and I simply didn't care. She tried numerous times to get my input on what plates to buy, what colors to paint the walls, and what color blankets I preferred. We eventually had a discussion where I told her that I honestly didn't care, as long as my PlayStation, TV and books remained in the house.

In retrospect I'm sad that I missed out on that, because I was involved in the nesting phase. Not so much the physical painting and assembling, but rather picking out a theme and finding stuff that goes with it. Even for a decor nihilist like myself, it was huge fun.

Imagination

As a writer, I have a fairly healthy imagination. This was probably my number one bonding experience. I imagined the idea of an entirely new person, experiencing all of the wonderful things life has to offer for the first time–ice cream, cartoons, the Marvel Cinematic Universe movies, motorized vehicles, and, eventually, beer. Like I said, dads tend to think about the baby as an older person with which they can share experiences. I couldn't wait to watch Jurassic Park with someone who hasn't seen it before. I'm still waiting. My wife thinks six is too early to watch Spielberg's masterpiece.

Use Your Hands

I'm not particularly good at this. Let me put it this way–I wouldn't sit, nor sleep on anything I built or assembled with my own hands.

I do have a friend who made everything from scratch in his garage–a cradle, rocking chair, closet, the works.

It's not even necessary to take it that far. A clay figurine, handmade necklace or candle will do the trick.

The basic idea is just another example of an item that's unique and special to the two of you.

Volunteer

I left this one for last, because it requires a strong stomach, and it's most definitely not for everyone.

As I mentioned near the beginning of the book, there's a shortage of fathers globally. In addition to the shortage, there's also a large number of children shunned by their dads because of their lifestyle choices. Fathers that choose to disavow their child because he/she is gay.

There's a massive need for attention from men globally, and you can volunteer to be one of those men.

I recommend volunteering to be a mentor, or a big brother to a child without a father. These projects are usually community-based, and are easy to find. The main aim is to spend time with these kids, teaching them skills that a father would normally teach, like how to change a tire, how to fix a bicycle, or how to fish. It goes deeper than that, however.

Like adults, kids have basic needs. One of those main needs is simply being noticed, and knowing that there's at least one person out there who cares.

I wouldn't recommend going this route if you don't have the time to fully commit, especially after your own child is born. Building a relationship with a child, and dumping them a few months later is cruel. The good news is that these projects are quite flexible, so you can find a way to work it into your life.

You can also volunteer to be a father for a day at the local school. There are various group activities in a year where parents are required. Schools will often send out notifications stating that they need volunteers to come cheer kids on, or help them with projects. It's just one day out of your life, and there's no long-term commitment.

I chose to volunteer for a project, though it did more damage than anything else. I was part of a group of men that drove to various hospitals with orphaned, terminally-ill kids. We thought we'd give them at least one day of joy in their short lives, which looked easier when planned on paper than it was in reality.

In reality you'd spend an hour or two handing over gifts, playing or reading with a specific child, and then move on. You get the contact details from the hospital to check in on the child later, only to find out that they had died.

I'm haunted to this day by those kids. I can't help but wonder how much potential the world lost. Could one of them have solved some large global issue? I take comfort in knowing that they at least had one day of joy. For an hour or two, they had the undivided attention of somebody who cared.

Sorry, I lied about the fatherhood statistics being the most depressing part of this book, but this really is the saddest it's going to get.

The idea is not to make you feel guilty for not partaking in some sort of charity. As I said in the first sentence, this isn't for everyone.

The idea is rather to get you to close this book, look around you and realize how blessed you are. Your wife may be a monster (more on that in the next chapter), but your baby is safe, well-fed and comfortable.

Keep that in mind every single day, even after they're born. There will be times when the baby is annoying, fussy, or quite simply a pain in the butt, but once everything has settled down, remember to be thankful that they are healthy, safe and loved.

Chapter 6: Life in the Third Trimester

One day you'll wake up and realize that your wife is missing. Somehow, somebody managed to swap her with a clone that's moodier, angrier and highly irritable.

We'll get to the reasons in a minute, but I'd like to give you some real-life examples of my battles with what I called the "hormone monster." Not to her face, for obvious reasons.

My wife would often fight with me shortly after I arrived home from work. "Why didn't you get *insert whatever item in here* at the store?" I was dumbstruck, because I didn't know I was supposed to. As it turns out, she'd often notice that we were running low on something, make a mental note to let me know to get it on the way home, and then forget about it. Even after I'd point this out, she'd be angry that I wasn't aware that *insert whatever item in here* was running low. This is a prime example of what's commonly referred to as "mommy brain."

Even my dream-self couldn't stay out of trouble. She once woke up, and told me that she had a dream about me. She wanted to go visit her mother, but I didn't want to take her because there was no money for gas. I was in no way involved, though I have to admit that my dream self sounds a bit like a cheapskate. Still, she hardly spoke to me that day, angry at a completely fictitious version of me that her subconscious had made up.

It's not all lows, however. Sometimes the mood swings the other way, in which case you'll be showered with compliments and affection. You'll spend the afternoon eating ice cream and watching Netflix, going to bed early to get those 10 hours.

At this point it's only fair to point out that not all women have these intense mood swings. During her second pregnancy, my wife was exponentially less aggravated.

To understand mood swings, and how to cope with them, we first need to look at the causes.

Why Is My Wife Acting This Way?

First off, let's just acknowledge the fact that there's no contest between what a woman goes through during pregnancy, and what a man goes through during pregnancy. As a man, you don't have something growing inside you, for example. Or think about the possibility of your penis being torn in a few short months. Those thoughts alone would make me grumpy, but it goes so much deeper than that.

According to Cari Nierenberg, in her article *Mood Swings & Mommy Brain: The Emotional Challenges of Pregnancy (2017)*, it's a mix of both biological and mental changes.

Mental Difficulties

Mood swings are most often credited to hormones. While hormones certainly play a role, there are various other underlying causes that result in mood swings.

The first mental difficulty is one you both likely share— fear. The same fears that keep you up at night are the same fears haunting her. It's a constant battle between knowing that you are prepared, and questioning whether you'll be a good parent.

In addition to wondering whether she'll be a good parent overall, she's also likely worried about breastfeeding, whether she'll suffer from postpartum depression, or that something might go wrong during the birth. Let's not forget about the prospect of having to push that baby out, or having major surgery.

Fear is not the only emotion she's dealing with. A pregnancy is like a daily assault of a hundred emotions, especially during the third and last trimester. Your wife will likely have a lot of time to reflect on her own childhood, which can be good or bad. If she's from a happy home, it will boost her confidence. An unhappy childhood will likely only add more fear to the mix. Will she be able to do a better job than her parents did?

And then the baby kicks, and she feels a sudden spurt of joy, followed by anxiety because that baby will soon be kicking around outside her body. That's a lot to go through in a space of just 10 minutes, so imagine how 12 waking hours must feel.

During my research, I also found many articles dedicated to body image issues during pregnancy. It's not something I ever thought of during my wife's two pregnancies. She was busy creating a human, so obviously she was going to get a bit bigger.

I asked my wife if she experienced any body image problems during and after the pregnancy, and she responded with a 'duh.'

These body image problems start way before pregnancy. It's a recurring theme in a woman's life. From a young age, women face a constant bombardment of unrealistic expectations. Beautiful, slim, tanned and big breasted women are plastered all over magazines, television, websites and social media. Anything less than that is simply not acceptable.

The same is true for pregnancy. My wife told me how angry she got whenever she paged through a magazine featuring a pregnant celebrity. They looked so happy, refreshed and completely unstressed. Then the baby would be born, and two weeks later their bodies look fit enough to take on the catwalk in Milan.

Biological Difficulties

The changes to a woman's body during pregnancy are massive. Blood volume increases, the immune system adapts to the baby, and the body starts releasing more hormones.

Both estrogen and progesterone levels increase by roughly 100 times the normal amount. The big offender is progesterone, which is also the hormone associated with premenstrual stress. Progesterone also increases anxiety if the woman already suffered from anxiety before the pregnancy.

The "mommy brain" is a combination of the above-mentioned hormones, fatigue and sleep deprivation. The short-term memory process is also affected, which explains why I was often in trouble for not buying things that I wasn't told I should buy.

There are various universities currently studying the brain during pregnancy, with some shocking results. The initial results showed a shrinking of the brain during the third and final trimester. Not by much, but noticeable. These studies have yet to provide conclusive findings, but the initial results are interesting.

Coping With Mood Swings

Simply understanding what your partner is going through is already a step in the right direction. Putting yourself in someone else's shoes leads to empathy, which you'll need to get through nine months of hormone overload.

With that in mind, we can look at some methods you can apply to ease your partner's burden.

Talk About Your Fears

We often don't share our fears with our partners, because we don't want to burden them with even more problems than they already have.

In this case, however, it's a bunch of shared fears. I'm willing to bet you that your partner feels inadequate in all the same ways you feel ill-equipped for the task ahead.

Talk about these fears, and do what you can to alleviate them.

Feeling stressed about the financial implications of having a baby? Sit down and work on a budget together to prove that you can afford it. And if you find out you can't, make the necessary changes in your lifestyle to get to the point where you can.

Not convinced you'll be decent parents? The fact that you're already worried about the child is proof that you're going to be a great parent. The only thing that should worry you is not worrying about the birth of a child.

Simply knowing that your partner is going through the same thing will already decrease stress levels. Have these conversations regularly, especially during the final months.

Accept The Emotional Rollercoaster

As discussed above, many of the fears are shared, but your wife has a number of additional fears to deal with. She not only faces the hormones, anxiety and pressures of the pregnancy, but most of what comes after.

The best you can do is accept the rollercoaster of emotions, and deal with them. Sometimes the anger aimed at you will be unfair, and in those instances it's best to just let it go. And, whatever you do, don't ever say the words, "it's just the hormones talking."

Burst The Body Image Bubble

A small compliment goes a long way, according to my wife. Even when it feels like you woke up next to Swamp Thing, it's worth saying that she looks even more beautiful today than yesterday.

It's also worth reminding your wife that models in pregnancy magazines and online articles probably went through two hours of makeup and preparation before the image was snapped.

As for how she looks after the birth, compared to how celebrities look, remind her that they probably have two assistants, three nannies and five personal trainers to help out around the house and get them back in shape. Us normal folk take a bit longer to get back to our former selves.

This tip is worth keeping in mind, even when your partner isn't expecting. Everyone loves to hear that they're looking good.

Don't Poke The Beast

When your wife is angry with you for not buying the milk and bread that she didn't tell you about on the way home, you can respond in two ways.

During her first pregnancy, I chose to defend myself. This only angered her more, which led to many awkward dinners. "I'd love to have some coffee right about now, but somebody forgot to buy milk," she'd say. I'd wonder what kind of passive-aggressive monster had replaced my wife.

There were also arguments about tiny, insignificant things that I don't even recall.

By the time the second pregnancy came around, I had learned my lesson. I phoned her on my way home to find out if there was anything we needed. I avoided unnecessary arguments by simply not getting dragged into them.

Chapter 7: Nesting

Nesting is a basic human instinct. It officially only happens a few weeks before the birth, and it's easy to spot the behavior. Once your wife starts cleaning the house, and throwing old stuff away, she's in the nesting phase.

The unofficial nesting phase happens long before that. That's when you start setting up the nursery.

Do dads nest? I'm not sure. I didn't nest the first time, but I most certainly did the second time. There are studies that suggest men do nest, if only to feel part of the process.

It makes sense in my case. I wasn't involved in setting up the nursery the first time, because I was away on a long trip. When we redid the nursery for my second child, we purposely waited for the December holidays so I could partake as well.

I'm a big fan of nesting, because it's prime bonding time. In the previous chapter I referred to talking openly and honestly about your fears, and most of our conversations happened while we were setting up the nursery.

The bonding experience even includes the baby. After the child is born, you can tell them that you were the one who put those shelves up. The baby won't understand, but you'll feel good about your contribution.

The Dad's Role

Nesting has two very distinct phases. The first is setting up the nursery, and getting all the things you need for the baby. The second phase happens near the end of the pregnancy. It's often described as a basic instinct that stems from our primal brains, but in reality it's nothing more than a mother ensuring that the house is clean, comfortable and safe.

As the dad, you get to play a role in both.

Setting Up The Nursery

My first nesting experience was completely different from the second.

My resounding memory of setting up the nursery during the first pregnancy is the amount of money it cost. I remember telling my wife that it feels like anything with the word 'baby' in it immediately receives a 30% markup. A normal dresser costs $100, while a baby dresser costs $130.

The first time you set up a nursery is expensive, if you buy new. All of the stuff I'm going to mention here is available second-hand as well, if you don't have a lot of budget.

A basic nursery requires a crib with a mattress, sheets and waterproof covers, a comfortable chair, dresser with drawers, baby monitor and the obvious items like clothes, diapers and wet wipes. Here's a top tip for you. You can never have enough wet wipes.

All in all, these basics cost us around $1,200. On the used market, you can easily reduce that by 50%. Instead of a baby monitor, you can use two old smartphones and a baby monitor app, for example.

In addition to the basics needed for the nursery, there are a few other things you require as well—a baby seat for the car, stroller and a transportable bed for the baby to sleep in when you're not at home.

The most important piece of advice I can give you is to stick to the basics mentioned above. The temptation to splurge on the latest baby gadgets is big. A salesperson will clock you as a newbie immediately, and will introduce you to the latest and greatest gadgets in babycare. More often than not, these gadgets are nothing more than a fad, so research what you need extremely well. I also recommend talking to other parents to find out what they used.

After our first outing, and after the baby tea, we ended up with a room full of the latest stuff. Around 90% of it was a nuisance, and added no value whatsoever. I can't recall 99% of the stuff, but I do remember a semi-upright chair with a vibrating function. We tried it once and it just wasn't upright enough for my son to see what was going on around him. The vibrating function just annoyed the heck out of him. We eventually just used his car seat as a seat around the house, and he was much happier in that.

Setting up the nursery the second time was much easier. We already had the basics, apart from a baby monitor. At age three, my firstborn decided to deposit the monitor's receiver in the toilet. I'm not sure whether it was a statement on the infringement of his privacy, or an accident. In any case, that's when we figured out that you can set up a much better, and more sensitive baby monitoring system with two old smartphones and an app. You also get a much clearer image of the room than you get on most modern monitors.

My involvement the second time around was more hands on. Some of it was good, some of it was bad.

I hated rebuilding all of the flatpack furniture, like the crib and the rocking chair. Here's a top tip: if you do buy flatpack stuff, store the instructions in a safe place. I had to rely on my intuition and building skills, which are basically non-existent. Let's just say that these items were put together using crude language more than anything else.

The part I loved was choosing a theme, and then decorating accordingly. My first born's theme was nautical, so this time we went for space. Instead of hiring people to paint for us, we did everything ourselves. Even my oldest, who was three years old at the time, pitched in where he could, handing me tools, and helping his mom cut stars out of cloth.

There were no decorations in the room that weren't hand made. The stars and clouds in front of the window were manufactured at our dining room table. I did the brunt of the painting, after which my wife painted a few clouds.

It was a magnificent bonding experience for the three of us, and the anticipation of the fourth member of our family was at an all-time high.

The Safety Phase

This is the instinctual phase of nesting, and it usually happens late in the pregnancy. More than anything, it's the final preparation for the arrival of the baby. Clothes get washed, clutter gets thrown away, every surface is scrubbed, and order is restored.

There are a few online tips on how you can help during this phase, but one is often left out. While the main focus is on getting the house ready for the baby, parents often forget about their own needs. So do yourself a favor and go to the grocery store and make sure that the cupboards and fridge are fully stocked. You won't get a lot of time to run errands during that first week, so be prepared. Don't forget to buy extra coffee, because a lot of people are going to come by to see the new baby.

While your wife is busy with the clothes, blankets, and cleaning, you can start with baby proofing the house. Once they start crawling, babies have a unique talent for finding the most dangerous objects in the house, and that's what you want to focus on.

I'm sorry to say that there's no life hack for baby proofing. You just have to get down on your knees and view every room from a baby's perspective. I didn't do this the first time, and I was alarmed at just how many sharp edges there are in a house. The only solution is to crawl around and look for possible hazards.

While you're at it, it's worth planning a few months in advance. Eventually that baby will learn how to stand up against things, and will then start digging in drawers. We found this out the hard way, while the three of us were in the kitchen. I was washing the dishes, and my wife was busy cooking. My oldest stood up against the kitchen drawers, honed in on the most dangerous one and opened it. Luckily we both caught him just before he could remove a sharp knife.

As you can see, it's not just about bumping into things. You also have to keep an eye out for things that could easily fall over, low drawers with dangerous things, and even something as innocent as a toilet. As I mentioned earlier, my son discovered the toilet quite early on, and had a habit of depositing things there. In addition to his baby monitor, he also threw the only key to our garage door in there. How did he get his hands on the key? As it turns out, our key holder was mounted too low down on the wall.

Chapter 8: The Big Day

Up until now you've probably had some life-changing days–graduating high school, getting a degree, buying your first car or house, and getting married. They all count as massive milestones, yet none of them will ever compare to this day.

How do I know that? Well, I've been through every one of the things listed above, and they all fade over time. I obviously remember the day I got married, because we celebrate the date every year, but as for the rest, I'm struggling to even attach a month.

I can give you an hour-by-hour lowdown of our big day. I can even tell you exactly what shirt I was wearing, and what I had for dinner that night.

But that's not what this chapter is about. It's rather about managing expectations, and the transformative moment you'll undoubtedly experience.

Birth Number One

By the time the big day arrives, a few things will be in place. As responsible parents, you'll already have a bag packed with everything mom and the baby will need for their stay in the hospital. You'll have a birth plan. My wife's birth plan was to do it naturally, followed by some skin-on-skin time. My plan was to be there, and do whatever the nurses told me.

As I mentioned in chapter 4, things didn't work out the way we planned. It all went a bit sideways, and my wife had to have an emergency C-Section.

What I didn't tell you is what happened after. It's a quick process, over and done within 15 minutes. After my son was inspected and weighed, he was handed over to me for a few seconds, so I could show my wife. I felt so bad for her, because she could do nothing but watch. Even so, she was thrilled.

A nurse took my son from me, put him in a climate-controlled box, and told me to follow her. I still wanted to check on my wife, but I was assured that she was doing perfectly fine, and that I was needed elsewhere.

As my son was pushed from the surgery room to the maternity ward, he passed his extended family for the first time. Unfortunately, there was no time to chat. The nurse was adamant that we keep moving. My mom was still trying to get the camera on her phone ready, but by that time we were gone.

In the maternity ward they placed him in an open crib under a warm light. And then we were left alone. The only two people in that entire ward. This left me with a massive moral conundrum.

On our way out to surgery, we passed our family for the first time. Because it was an emergency, I couldn't tell them much more than it was an emergency and I had to go. Now I was back, both mom and baby were safe, but I had no way of communicating with my family. I felt I needed to at least let my wife's mom know that she was fine. But I had a problem. I was now dressed in hospital scrubs. My clothes and all my personal belongings–including my phone–were stuck somewhere in a locker. I had no way of communicating with the outside world.

While all of these thoughts were playing around in my head, I was also busy introducing myself to my son. I held out a finger to touch his hand, and he grabbed it. He must have recognized my voice, because he was oddly calm for a person who had just entered the realm of the living less than an hour ago.

I knew I could not leave his side, but I desperately wanted to let my wife's mom know that she was perfectly fine, and around an hour behind us.

I couldn't yell for fear of scaring the baby, but I had to get the attention of the nurses just around the corner. Using some impressive Spider-Man-like skills, I somehow managed to keep my finger in my son's hand, while sticking a foot out the door and wiggling it for some attention.

One of the nurses came running, and I asked her to please just tell the family outside that everything was fine.

Eventually my wife was rolled back into her room, after which we were told we could join her. I rolled my son down the hall to officially meet his mother. They fit together perfectly. It was almost as if the space above her folded arms was tailor-made just for him.

All was quiet for an hour or so, but then the baby started wriggling around. Thanks to the baby classes, I knew to expect that first meconium poop. This sticky, almost black substance is made up of cells, fat and protein. It doesn't smell bad, but it is your first chance to try your hand at changing a diaper. I'm happy to report that I not only changed that diaper, but the clothing as well. I wasn't grossed out at all. I would go to the ends of the earth to ensure my child was happy, so changing a nappy didn't seem like such a big deal.

Soon after both of them fell asleep, and I sat there quietly until the nurses told me visiting hours for fathers was over. I left there with an uncomfortable knot in my stomach, knowing that I was leaving what was most dear to me behind in that hospital room.

Oddly enough, I nearly ended up in the hospital that same night. While I was at the hospital, my mom was kind enough to go drop a pizza at home for me. She locked the gate, not knowing that I didn't have any keys on my then brand-new Subaru's keys yet. The main house key was back at the hospital, but I wasn't fazed. I knew how to break into my own house, so I'd just do that, find the spare keys on the inside and open the gate. As I reached the top of the wall, one of the bricks came loose, and I fell face forward into the small garden on the other side. Luckily, nothing was broken. Thank heavens for that.

Our first birthing plan certainly didn't include all of us being in the hospital at the same time.

Birth Number Two

Armed with the knowledge that birthing plans rarely work out, we decided on a straight-forward one for our second child.

Natural births are not recommended after a woman's already had a C-Section, so that was decided for us. Unlike the first time, we knew the exact date, and what time to report.

If anything, this day was extremely dull. We had to be there early morning, but the surgery was only scheduled late in the afternoon. All we had to do was wait.

The main difference between this birth and the previous one was that it wasn't an emergency. My second son was born late afternoon, and once again I spent an hour with him in the hospital's nursery. Since our last visit, some upgrades have been made. One of these upgrades was a viewing window into the nursery, so my family could at least get a look at baby number two.

He was born in time for visiting hours, but we decided in advance that only one visitor would be allowed that day. We wanted to introduce our oldest to his new brother. It was a magical moment, etched into my memory forever.

I managed to get in bed that night without falling down a wall. I wasn't alone this time either. My oldest was with me, and as we lay in bed that night I asked him if he had any questions. "Just one," he said.

"Are we going to keep him?"

The Big Lesson

I told you both stories, because I want to make a point. It's all fine and dandy to have a plan, in fact, I encourage it. It keeps the nerves down as you get closer to the big day.

The plan may work out perfectly, as it did with my second son. Or it may not, as it did with my first.

The point is that it just doesn't matter. At the end of the day the only thing that matters is a healthy mom and a healthy baby. How you get there is irrelevant.

It may seem unlikely if you're the kind of person who likes to be in control at all times, but trust me on this. The moment they hand you that baby, it's like a switch that activates.

The best way I can think of describing it is like having a volume button for life. That baby just turns the volume down on everything else. You suddenly realize that nothing you deemed important before will ever matter as much as that child. Apart from your relationship with your spouse, that is.

Take Care of Your Relationship

To say that a baby puts strain on a relationship is the understatement of the century. Some of the most stressful days of your life lie ahead, and you may as well make peace with that now. It is inevitable, no matter how strong your bond is.

And your relationship with your significant other is worth saving, because you still have to spend a lifetime with each other. At some point the kids will grow up and leave the house, and if you don't look after your relationship constantly, you'll be left behind with a stranger.

What Causes The Strain?

In my experience, there are three main contributors to the strain. This is in addition to the crying and paranoia I'll be discussing in the next chapter.

The first is a lack of enough time. Before the baby came along, your time was your own. You could watch a movie at 2:00 p.m. on a Saturday, because you're an adult and you get to do what you want. If you wanted to sleep until 11:00 a.m. the next morning, nothing was standing in your way.

Then there's the shared time with your wife. Before the baby, you ate dinner together in front of the television. You spend Saturdays walking around naked in the house, because why not. On Sundays you went for an agreeable brunch, and took an afternoon nap.

You can kiss all of that goodbye.

Let me give you a rundown of an average day in our house. We all wake up at 6:00 a.m., have breakfast, get dressed, and head off in our various directions. We all meet up again at the house at around 5:00 p.m., at which point I spend an hour playing with the kids. At 7:00 p.m. it's bath time, followed by dinner at 7:30 p.m. Bedtime is at 8:00 p.m. By the time my wife and I have had a bath, it's 9:00 p.m., and we're both too tired to do anything. Sex? Forget about it. If you're lucky, you'll watch one episode of a show on *Netflix* before falling into a coma.

Over time this builds resentment. You never have any time alone with your wife, not to mention any time just by yourself.

We already touched on the second contributor, which is an all-new element being introduced into your already fully-functioning lives. To accommodate the needs of the baby, who is now the most important member of the household, massive sacrifices have to be made. Since we were both in the media, traveling for work on a weekly basis, we knew one of us had to give up work. My wife did it out of her own free will, deciding she'd rather raise her own kids than have somebody else do it for us.

This leads us to the biggest contributor to strain on the relationship: not understanding what the other person goes through on a daily basis. I was convinced I was working the hardest, in the same way she was convinced there was no way I could possibly be working as hard as she was.

It was uncharacteristically selfish behaviour from both our sides. The truth is that we were both taking serious strain. She spent the day with the baby, handing it over to me as soon as I arrived home. I resented her for this, because I also spent the day working, and in my mind I also deserved a short break.

How To Ease The Strain

I find it best to rip that Band-Aid right off, and speak honestly about how I'm feeling. My wife knows to do the same with me whenever something is bothering her.

That's how we solved the biggest problem we had, which was thinking that each of us was working harder than the other.

I explained to her that I spent an hour in traffic in the morning, eight hours at work and another hour in traffic on the way home. She then ran me through her schedule, which was basically being responsible for a baby when he was awake, and then cleaning, and cooking when he wasn't. We were both working hard, and there was no solution. Sometimes you just have to suck it up, and stand in for your partner. You may think your tank is running on empty, but you'd be surprised at what you can achieve.

Pushing yourself to the boundaries constantly isn't healthy either, so don't be afraid to ask for help. Our son was around four weeks old when we decided to take a short break from him. My mother came over to babysit while we went out. Nothing fancy, just a quick ice cream at McDonald's. We lasted around 25 minutes before the separation anxiety kicked in, and we went home. Even so, those 25 minutes alone was enough to recharge the batteries for a few weeks. The separation anxiety also dissipates as time goes by. I'm happy to report that we can now leave our kids with the grandparents for a whole two days.

You also need to recognize when your partner is on edge, and when a break is in order. Give her a few hours off to do whatever, and she'll do the same for you.

Finally, it's worth taking stock of what you have. Instead of focussing on not getting any sleep, being annoyed with the change in your lifestyle, and resenting your partner for not doing enough, focus on all the good things.

You have a beautiful baby, a roof over your head, food in the fridge, and at least two people who love and adore you.

I'm the first to admit that it's pretty hard to focus on the above when it's 3:00 a.m. in the morning, your shirt is full of vomit stains, and the baby is trying his/her best to burst your eardrums, but it's worth a shot.

You might think that these relationship issues will only last for as long as the baby is small, but they'll be with you for as long as the child is in the house. Trust me, I know. My two boys are way beyond that initial crying phase, yet they still have a way of dominating your entire life.

And the truth of the matter is that one day they'll be big, and won't live under your roof anymore. Not only will you miss them, but you'll be living with someone you've been resenting for 20 years.

By all means, do your utmost to ensure the safety, comfort and health of your baby, but always make time for your relationship. Never allow yourself to get to a place where you're simply staying together for the kids.

Statistics have shown that the divorce rate skyrockets in the 50+ age group due to empty nest syndrome. I'm not there yet, but I can only imagine what it must feel like to have dedicated all that time to the kids, only to be left behind with a stranger.

Keep the above in mind whenever you drop the kids at your parent's place for a weekend away, and the guilt will quickly drop away.

Chapter 9: The First Few Weeks With Baby

The first few days are extremely underwhelming. The average newborn sleeps between 14 to 17 hours per day, only waking for feeding time. When this happens, you feed them, burp them, and change their diaper. Then they go back to sleep. Some light crying might happen in between, but nothing too drastic.

They continue this routine long enough to lure you into a false sense of parenting success. Just when you think you've got this, they turn six weeks old and unleash their full crying potential. Though it differs from baby to baby, experts reckon the most crying happens between week six through to week eight. During that time, they spend an average of three hours per day crying. Colicky babies cry even more, even though there's absolutely nothing wrong with them.

The big problem is a lack of communication. At six weeks old, their needs may be more than just a feeding, and there's absolutely no way of telling what that is, other than crying. By month four you should be able to tell from their facial expressions, but that still leaves you with three months of not knowing what to do.

The first piece of advice people normally give you is to remain calm. I'm not going to do that, because you won't be able to. You're a first-time parent with no idea what to do, with a constantly crying baby providing the background noise. Chances are, you're also mad at your wife, and she's mad at you too. If somebody had come up to me during those midnight crying sessions, and told me to remain calm,

I would have punched them. The good news is that it is so much easier the second time around, but you won't know that yet.

Why Is The Baby Crying?

We struggled with our first child, not always sure what to do. I'd suggest that maybe he was still hungry, while my wife was sure he was struggling to pass gas. The result was conflict between us, and I'm sure that tension transferred through to the baby as well.

Somehow we managed to survive the first three months with our marriage intact. To ensure it wouldn't happen again with our second son, we talked about the first three months at great length before we got to that stage.

Armed with the experience from our first child, we compiled a list of the most likely causes for crying. Then we simply started from the top and worked our way down. This worked 99% of the time.

As a new dad, you can use this list to do the same. I'm not going to tell you to remain calm, but work your way through it and see what happens. After a while you might even see a pattern emerging, which means you can solve the problem before it even happens.

The Baby Is Hungry

Breastfeeding a baby is extremely difficult. In the beginning they have problems latching, it hurts, and you're never quite sure how much they've had to drink. This was our main struggle, because we'd be under the impression that he had enough once he fell asleep. Shortly after he'd be awake again, crying for more. By then your assumption is that it's something else, so you start searching for the cause. Meanwhile, the little guy is lying there screaming for more milk.

The crying got so bad that we eventually took him to the doctor. He was weighed and they found that he was slightly under the expected growth curve. His weight wasn't ideal either.

My wife wasn't producing enough milk, so we had to switch over to formula. Our lives improved drastically from this point on. We knew exactly how much he needed, and we could control the intake. If he fell asleep during the feeding, and the bottle was still half full, we knew he wasn't done.

The easiest way to tell when a baby is full is to see how he/she reacts to the breast or bottle. If they're disinterested, distracted by something else, or sleepy, chances are they're full.

While we're on the topic of feeding, don't ever be smug about breastfeeding. Yes, science has proven that it's the absolute best, and yes, there are parents out there who do it for convenience. But labeling all non-breastfeeding mothers as irresponsible and lazy is uncalled for. Think twice before you share your opinions on breastfeeding the next time you're in the company of other parents.

The Baby Is Gassy

There's still some debate around this topic. Many people believe that passing gas is too routine to cause a baby any discomfort, but I respectfully disagree. Too many times have I rubbed out a burp, only for the baby to settle down immediately for a few hours.

I don't mean to brag, but I'm a bit of a burp master. I seem to have the golden touch when it comes to rubbing out winds.

There are various methods you can use–holding the baby over your shoulder and patting him/her on the back, laying them down on your lap while also patting, but the method that works best for me is leaning back on a chair, while laying the baby's stomach down on my chest. I then rub the back from the bottom to the top a few times. Works like a charm.

It worked on both my sons, but you might find one of the other methods more effective.

Dirty Diaper

This is worth checking at least once an hour, because diaper rash is serious business.

It's a mistake you only make once. Rubbing bum cream on the sore bum of a baby that doesn't understand why you're hurting him/her requires skill and patience.

Checking for a dirty diaper without waking the baby also requires serious skill. When it's summer and the baby is wearing nothing more than a vest, it's easy as pie. During the winter months, when multiple layers are involved, it's not as easy.

I learned fairly quickly that it's easier to simply carefully maneuver a finger through the various layers of clothing, and then sticking your finger in the side of the diaper. A method closely resembling the way you'd check the oil level in your car. It's gross, but trust me, it gets much grosser than that in the coming months.

I found the smelling the bum method to be unreliable. More often than not, it was just a lingering wind, which you only found out once the baby was fully awake and undressed.

Too Hot, Too Cold

Another topic that my wife and I used to argue about constantly. She read somewhere that the appropriate number of layers is whatever the parent is wearing, plus one additional layer for the baby.

She's also extremely sensitive to cold weather, so the moment the temperature dipped beneath 70, she'd layer the baby to the point where he couldn't move his arms.

Babies are extremely sensitive to temperature, so if any of the above methods don't work, try adding or removing some layers.

Tired

Yup. Just like us, babies get cranky when they're tired. The main problem here is that it's not something you'd suspect, given how easily they fell asleep during the first few weeks. Getting them to sleep requires more effort in the later months.

My recommendation is to get them to sleep in a room where there's as little stimulation as possible. A simple rocking motion should be more than sufficient to ease them off to dreamland.

While we're on the topic, I noticed a trend whenever visitors came over. Everybody wants to hold the baby at some point, and interact with him/her. This is a lot of stimulation for a baby younger than three months.

My sons were extremely cranky after family visits, and it would take a long time to get them to settle down. I asked a doctor friend about it, and she confirmed that it's quite easy to overstimulate a baby, but that it was not just that. Their bodies are also highly sensitive, which can lead to aches and pains after being passed around the room like a football.

You can keep this from happening by sticking to the baby's routine, regardless of whether there are visitors or not. It might come across as rude, but we had strict rules about who could handle the baby and for how long. And when it was feeding or sleeping time, we stuck to the schedule. Your guests may be offended, but they're not the ones who are going to be stuck with a fussy, screaming baby later that day.

Just A Cuddle

Sometimes, a baby just wants to be held. It spent nine months in a confined, warm space, and a nice, warm cuddle is the next best thing.

Swaddling works like a charm, but only on certain babies. That's when you wrap them up tightly in a blanket, so their arms can't move. And then you hold them tightly to your chest.

My oldest loved swaddling, but my youngest absolutely hated it. He would get furious when he couldn't move his arms freely.

When To Call The Doctor

This is tough advice to give, because I don't know your child, and 90% of this requires knowing your child.

Trust me on this. As a parent, you'll know when something is off. The baby will look and act differently. I think one also develops a sort of sixth sense about these things.

The fact of the matter is this: when you're a first-time parent, you'll be visiting the doctor's office way more than you should. Some people feel ashamed about going to the doctor, not wanting to waste his/her time on something as simple as a runny nose. You have to weigh those feelings up against the discomfort of having a sick child, which means everything to you.

I had no qualms about going to the emergency room whenever a fever struck, or I felt like something was wrong. I always apologized to the doctor if it was something completely harmless, but they were never concerned.

As one doctor told me, "when it comes to babies, it's better to feel like an idiot for coming in for something minor, than waiting a few days for it to turn into something major."

My Paranoid Phase

One of the reasons I'm such a big fan of baby classes is that it's presented by people who know babies. They've dedicated their lives to studying pediatrics, which makes them the number one source of information.

Sure, it's a good idea to do additional reading, but keep a close eye on the sources. I don't claim to be an expert. I'm merely just a dad with two kids, sharing an experience.

Because I'm a curious person by nature, I did as much reading as I could, even though the nurse who lectured us told us not to delve too deep into certain topics. In other words, don't go down the rabbit hole when it comes to all the bad things that can happen.

The one bad thing that got stuck in my mind was Sudden Infant Death Syndrome (SIDS). Science doesn't have a proper explanation for why it happens, but a baby basically just stops breathing during the night.

It's also the number one topic that pops up when you specifically search for things that can go wrong. Now, before we go any further, let me put your mind at ease. Each year around four million babies are born in the USA. Of those, roughly 2,500 die as a result of SIDS. That means your baby has a 0.06% chance of dying of SIDS.

There are also numerous ways you can lower that percentage even more by putting the baby to sleep on his back on a firm mattress. Other tips are just basic common sense, like not smoking around the baby.

Still, even with all this information at my disposal, and knowing all the methods for preventing SIDS, I couldn't help but worry.

For the first six months, our son slept in our room in a Moses Cradle next to the bed. I had an extremely tough time falling asleep, constantly worrying about SIDS. I'd read for an hour or so, walk over to check the baby by holding a small mirror up to his nose, and then try to settle down. After struggling for 30 minutes, I'd get up again to check the baby. I'd repeat this routine at least three times until I eventually fell asleep. Some night I'd wake up at 3:00 a.m., horrified that the baby's breathing hadn't been checked for a few hours.

There are baby monitors that go as far as monitoring breathing, but once you Google them, it won't take you long to stumble across the tragic story of a baby that got tangled up in all the cables necessary for this particular system.

I'd love to tell you that I was less anxious the second time around, but that wouldn't be true. I followed the same routine, until they were around six months old and out of the SIDS danger zone.

Even now that they're six and three years old, I still go into their rooms every night before I go to bed to hear them breathing.

I sincerely hope that I didn't frighten you with this section, because that was not the intent. It's rather meant to demonstrate how we tend to get fixated on tragedies instead of success stories.

It's even more relevant in the age of social media, because everything you read online results in targeted advertising on social media. The more horror stories you read, the more content and advertising you'll get to remind you of them.

I have a tactic I use whenever I get paranoid, which is quite often. I'm extremely scared of flying, so it only made sense that I chose a career that involved at least four flights a week during my younger years. It got so bad that I eventually went to a psychiatrist for help, and he cured me in one session by simply changing the way I think.

As anxious human beings, we're always more focused on what could go wrong. Every time I got on a plane, I was sure the engine would blow up as soon as we were in the air, in the same way I'd imagine the baby not breathing when I got to his bedside. Statistically, the chances of both scenarios are extremely slim, but it didn't stop me from constantly thinking about it.

I offer that advice to you now, in all its beautiful simplicity. Instead of imagining the plane going down in a ball of flames, rather imagine it gliding through the air safely and touching down at the end destination softly and smoothly. The same can be applied to the baby. Rather than imagining the worst, imagine waking up the next morning and having a wonderful breakfast with the family.

I know it sounds stupid, but I promise you it works.

Chapter 10: Setting Boundaries

For decades it has been the accepted norm that one of the grandparents would come live in the house for the first few weeks to help out with the newborn.

I'm not a fan of this tradition, for various reasons. As I mentioned in the previous chapters, there will already be more than enough stress to go around, so why would you want to add to that by inviting another outsider into the mix?

The main reason we used to do this is simply traditional gender roles. Dad would return to work as soon as possible, and mom would stay home with the baby. By the time dad got home, the baby had to be bathed, dinner had to be cooked, and the day's paper should have been waiting next to dad's favorite chair, right next to his slippers. Had I tried this with my wife, she would have burned my chair, and hit me with the newspaper until I realized that the child was my responsibility as well.

Having said that, there are laws in other countries that are horribly outdated. Here in the USA it's still not perfect, but it at least allows for a decent amount of time off, even though you don't get paid for it. The law states that you may take 12 weeks of unpaid leave, backed up by job protection. While you won't be earning anything during that time, you at least have a job to go back to. Hopefully you find out about the pregnancy sooner rather than later, which means you can start working on a savings account as soon as possible.

There are many reasons you want to set healthy boundaries going forward, starting with the massive change in family dynamics.

New Parents Dealing With Their Parents

To me, this was one of the hardest parts of becoming a dad. You have to walk a fine line between protecting your own brand-new family, and the feelings of your old family. And by that, I mean you need to know when to tell your parents when to back off.

There's already an inherent problem in that the baby is the culmination of two families coming together. What are the chances that these two families had the same habits, rules, beliefs and hobbies?

My wife and I are a prime example of two very different families coming together. My wife was raised in a religious, middle-class, and strict environment. I was raised non-religious, in an upper-class suburb, and I'll admit that my parents spoiled me a bit. I basically got everything I wanted.

Our biggest clash wasn't about religion, as you'd expect. I think religion is a beautiful thing, and we happen to belong to an all-inclusive church that teaches both adults and children to respect everyone, regardless of their race or sexual orientation. That particular hurdle was easy to cross.

The little things were much harder. I'd happily buy my kids whatever they wanted, while my wife was more pragmatic. They both first had to understand the value of things, not to mention that teaching them that you can't always get what you want from an early age is not a bad idea.

My wife and her family also had dinner at a table every night, talking about their day and bonding. On our side, you could have dinner in front of the television, or in your room. We had our own way of bonding, and my parents never pushed the idea of having family dinners.

Between these two vastly different upbringings, you have to find a compromise. It's not that difficult when it's just you and your partner, and you can talk openly and honestly about the things you feel strongly about. I don't particularly care about where I eat dinner, so it was easy to get into the habit of eating dinner at a table. Not being able to give my sons presents was a bit harder, but my wife got me to slow down a bit.

But throw in two sets of parents, who have already successfully raised their own kids using their own methods, and you have the recipe for a perfect storm. Especially when one of the grandparents has a degree in child psychology, like my mother in law.

It also didn't help that our son was the first grandchild on both sides of the family, so it was a big event for all involved.

The big problem is that there's this huge family dynamic shift. Parents being parents, they still feel that they have some sort of control over your life. My mum would always give me some money whenever I went over for a visit, even though I had a well-paying job. She knew this, so I'm guessing it was just some sort of method to at least make her feel like she was contributing to my life in some way.

I respect both sets of parents, as I'm sure you do. But here's the thing: Raising kids is all about finding what works for your own unique family setup. You have a right to screw things up in your own distinctive way, and to learn from that. And if your parents say they never messed up, they're lying.

Why Set Boundaries?

As I mentioned earlier, it's nearly impossible to give advice in this regard, because every family is different. While I struggled with the above, you might have another set of problems you have to deal with.

The one thing all parents have in common is the mammoth descent of visitors to come see the new baby. I fully understand that it's a big deal, and that everyone is excited about the latest member of the family, but consider the already heavy burden your wife is carrying through this phase.

As I said in the first chapter, there will be enormous strain on both of you. In addition to still learning what the baby requires at any given time, you will be tired, probably angry at each other, and still very much in shock that this giant responsibility is now here, and not going away anytime soon. Do you really want to invite visitors over to come witness the suffering?

Visitors will no doubt be aware of the circumstances, but you'll still feel a need to entertain them in some way. They'll also each want to hold the baby at some point, which I have a problem with for two reasons. First, it messes with building a routine. Getting that baby into a routine as soon as possible should be your number one priority, as it's one of the things that will help you retain some semblance of sanity. But then visitors arrive, pass the baby along like it's a bong, and that routine goes down the drain. They get to leave after a few hours, but you're the one stuck with an overtired infant trying his/her best to match an aircraft's decibel reading.

The second reason I don't like visitors has to do with health. During our baby classes, we learned that babies are extremely susceptible to viruses and such, since they don't have an immune system yet. The first thing most people want to do with the new baby is hold it and kiss it all over. It seems harmless, but that's far from the case. We were told that an unfortunately large percentage of babies end up back in hospital with whooping cough or influenza because of this.

Not that I needed another reason to keep my kids from kissing extended family members. I hated family reunions as a child. Once a year the entire extended family would get together, and my brother and I would have to march from one old lady to the next, kissing them as we went along. My mother enforced this law, backed-up by my grandmother, also keeping a watchful eye ensuring that no far along family member went without a kiss. Back then, being a rebellious seven-year-old, I made a mental note to never force my own kids to kiss anyone they didn't want to.

Sure enough, the result was a large family fight, but I stood my ground. They were my kids after all, and I was allowed to make the rules. This rule is now more relevant than ever considering that we just went through a once in a lifetime pandemic. I stand firmly by it, and whenever a member of the family tries to get my boys to kiss whomever,

I don't hesitate to intervene, even if it means somebody's feelings get hurt. I usually take the time to explain my choice, and, to be honest, most people respect it. But there is some pushback from older generations who believe kissing is a sign of respect.

The other big fallout we had was during the festive season. Where would the baby spend his first December holiday, and with whom? The moment the parents started talking this way, my wife and I devised a plan. To ensure there wouldn't be any jealousy from either side, we'd have Christmas at our house, and we'd invite both sides of the family.

This was an exhausting affair, and an expensive one at that. But it is the best way to ensure that everyone gets to see the baby over the festive season, so it's a tradition we're keeping. I find the jealousy between grandparents extremely strange. It's almost as if they have a stopwatch, keeping track of every second one of my kids spends time at the other grandparents' house. And then they want the exact same amount of time. It's one of those odd things in life. You have kids, and all of a sudden, your parents start behaving like kids as well.

Finally, there's a huge generation gap between us and our parents when it comes to health. In the appointments following the birth of a baby, they take all sorts of measurements to ensure that he/she is following the recommended growth curve. When the time comes for solids, you're given an expertly researched diet to follow.

My wife was extremely serious about sticking to this plan, and who could blame her. It was designed by people much smarter than us. People who have dedicated their lives to studying baby eating habits and nutrition.

Yet, in waltzes my mother, wondering why the baby is still on milk. "Back when my son was young, he was already on maize," she said. Besides maize not being that easy to digest, we already had a freezer full of organic vegetables, boiled and smashed, ready to be eaten when the time comes.

I swear she tried to give him a piece of chocolate when he was just two weeks old. Thank goodness for modern feeding plans and access to information. Back in the day it seems they just went with whatever method was passed on from the previous generation. And the generation before that.

And don't even get me talking about home remedies. My firstborn had some trouble with teething, which kept us up for a few nights. We soldiered on until we needed a break from the screaming and the not sleeping. It was time to call for backup, so grandma packed her bags and came to the rescue.

Before we left for the hotel, we gave her strict instructions on the feeding schedule, as well as the teething medicine. It was just a simple ointment, applied directly to the gums. It deadens the pain for a bit, but nothing too serious.

Arriving back the next day, the house was quiet. It seems grandma took one look at this newfangled ointment and decided that an old recipe handed down over the generations would do a better job. In her defense, the baby was sleeping better than he had in weeks.

"Finally," I thought. "There is some merit to these old homemade remedies after all."

Until it was my turn to give it to the baby. That tiny spoon of liquid knocked the wind out of him, and he gave the same sort of grimace you see on the face of someone who just drank a shot of moonshine. So, I tried it myself and there it was. The unmistakable taste of alcohol. No wonder the little guy was sleeping so soundly.

I phoned my mom asking her what the magic ingredients to this wonderful potion was. "Oh, you know, just the usual. Some sugar, some pain and fever medicine and a shot of whisky."

Sigh.

How to Set Boundaries

The important thing to remember is that all of the above comes from a good place. It's all done out of love, misguided it may be. Ask yourself, would you rather have the alternative? Parents that aren't involved or interested, or perhaps not even there anymore…

Whenever I feel overwhelmed by my parents' need to get involved in my affairs, I remind myself that I'm still their child, and that they're just trying to look out for me in the same way that I'm looking out for my sons.

I'll be the first to admit that I reacted too strongly to certain things, but I was exhausted and hadn't had the time to consider the above yet. The good news is that with age comes wisdom, which means it was much easier to set boundaries the second time around.

The first step to setting boundaries is to decide what those boundaries should be. There are families who are extremely close, and don't mind when somebody pops up uninvited. We're not like that. We like our privacy very much, so our boundaries may seem a bit over the top to some. But luckily there is a way to set strict boundaries without burning bridges.

The first step is to realize what I mentioned above. The overbearing attention, hints, and advice don't come from a bad place. They're not trying to tell you that you're a bad parent from the start. They have experience, and they want to impart that knowledge to make your life easier. Never forget that your parents will always have your back.

That's why my first piece of advice is to actually listen to their fears, because underneath it all there will be a positive intention.

I'll explain with an example. We were absolutely resolute in our decision to never allow co-sleeping in our house. That's when you allow a toddler to climb into bed with you, instead of sleeping in their own bed. For obvious reasons, you should never do it with a baby. But around two years of age, when they can get out of their own bed and walk to yours, they'll want to sleep with you.

We were adamant that we'd never allow it, to protect the solitude of our own room. It sounded like a good plan, right until a toddler climbs into your bed at 3 a.m. in the morning in the winter, and you simply can't work up the energy to take them back to bed. It's a bit like promising yourself that you'll never bribe your kids with candy, and before you know it, you're offering a candy bar as a reward for cleaning a room.

My mother was concerned that we'd smother the child, but since he was two years old already, there was little chance of it happening.

I let her explain her fears to me, and I listened. I then told her how I felt, not wanting to drag a child back to their bed in the dead of winter, lying there waiting for them to get back to sleep, only to tiptoe back to my own bed.

We met somewhere in the middle. I recognized her fears, and told her that my number one concern was also my kids' safety. I'd never do anything to put them in harm's way. That way we shared a common concern, rather than battling pointlessly over conflicting points of view.

Chapter 11: The First Year With Baby

Here's some good news for you: if you can make it through the first three months, you can easily handle the rest.

For the rest of the first year, there are only two things I recommend you look out for. The first is when they learn that they can put things in their mouth. They will put anything, and I really do mean everything, into their mouth. The second thing is crawling. Babies have absolutely zero sense of self-preservation and will crawl at top speed everywhere. Under tables, over dogs, downstairs, straight into the emergency room. We'll look at some more milestones later on in this chapter.

In this chapter I first want to cover some of my misadventures in parenting.

Throughout this book, I've given you examples from my own life. I wanted it to be as relatable as possible, because you will make mistakes. I made plenty. At the time they weren't funny, but I can look back at them now and laugh out loud, and hope you do too.

Misadventures In Parenting

I want to tell you three stories. The first is not meant to be funny, but rather to demonstrate how quickly things can go wrong. I like to think of myself as an extremely responsible parent, but I messed up. I beat myself up mentally for weeks after the incident, until my wife finally told me that I was just human.

The second story is about listening to your wife. As men we tend to think we know everything, but here's the truth fellas: we don't. If your wife gives you baby advice, listen to it.

The third is the grossest thing that ever happened to me as a parent. I want to share it with you, so you know exactly what you're getting into.

Our First ER Visit

As babies get older, they get more animated and stronger. Remember to enjoy the days when you put them down and they stay exactly where you put them, because the moment they become mobile, the metaphorical poop hits the fan.

On this particular occasion I had just finished bathing my son. I wrapped him up in a towel and put him on his changing station. It was slightly higher than the average table, so you don't need to bend over every time you need to change a diaper.

He was squirming and bouncing up and down on the table, so I kept one hand on his belly to keep him in place, while I rummaged around in the drawer to find a diaper. I soon discovered we were out of diapers, which meant I had to open the cupboard directly below the shelf to open a new pack.

My wife was in the room with us, sitting in the comfortable chair, and taking a short break. After a long day of taking care of our son, I wasn't going to disturb what had likely been the most comfortable moment of her day.

I forgot what I was doing for a second and removed my other hand from the baby's belly, and reached for the closet below.

The next thing I heard was an ear-piercing shriek, and I reacted immediately. I caught the baby mid-air with one hand before he hit the floor. But for some reason, his mouth was bleeding, and it wouldn't stop.

We got in the car, rushed to the emergency room, all the while thinking that we were going to get locked up for being irresponsible parents.

Funny enough, by the time we got to a doctor, the bleeding had stopped. I told him what happened, thinking he was going to tell me that the bleeding was a result of some brain injury.

He took my son, opened his mouth and said, "yup, just as I thought."

As it turns out, it was something he had seen a thousand times before. Babies have a small piece of skin on the inside of their mouths between the back of the upper lip and the gums. It tears quite easily, and is notorious for bleeding a lot.

Just to be sure, he inspected the rest of the baby, but all he could find was a red imprint of my right hand across his chest. "That probably won't leave a bruise, but just keep an eye on it."

This incident brought me right back down to earth. I let my guard down for a second, and we ended up in the emergency room.

Poop In My Pocket

This story finds us in the exact same location as the story before, but a few months later, and right before bedtime.

I was busy changing a diaper, but this time my wife was standing next to me. We were having a chat about something insignificant, when she interrupted me.

"He's not done pooping yet. I can see it in his face," she said.

"There's no way there's still anything left," I told her as I looked down at the mess below. Feeling confident that his small body simply didn't have enough space to accommodate any more poop, I lifted up his legs to begin wiping.

The result was projectile pooping. Yes, my friend, I kid you not. You've probably heard about projectile vomiting and babies, but this is also a thing.

It came out in a majestic arc, missed the changing table completely, but ended up in my nightgown's pocket. If I didn't know any better, you'd think he was aiming for it.

The white nightgown was a write-off.

Always listen to your wife.

The Grossest Thing Ever

Once again we're in the same location, but this time I'm all by myself in the middle of the night.

It started out as a routine feeding, but soon escalated to a serious vomiting session. By the end it was all over me, all over him, on the chair, and on the floor. Nothing too serious, and nothing that hasn't happened before.

By that time I had built up a resistance to vomiting, as will you. You simply sit there and take it, let him get it all out.

This time, however, he was fairly amused by what he did, giving me a goofy smile as I glanced down at his face. What he did next was unforgivable, and one day when he's a man, I will get him back for it. I'm not sure how, but I still have more than a decade to figure it out.

I returned his smile, and made some friendly baby noises. In return he took his hand, which was drenched in vomit, and forced it into my mouth.

The noises I made while trying to swallow down the contents of my own stomach was enough to wake my wife up. She walked into the room, looked at the scene in front of her and gave me an inquiring glance.

I told her what happened and her response was not what I was expecting. Instead of showing some sympathy, or taking the baby so I could remove myself from the pool of chunder, she laughed so hard that she had to sit down on the floor.

She helped me eventually, but, like my son, I'm still plotting my revenge.

Big Milestones

If you subscribe to a weekly newsletter, you'll know what to look out for on any given week, but just in case, I added some of my favorites here. For the record, I kept track of baby development on Parents.com, which gives you a thorough breakdown of what to expect in the article, *Baby Milestones Chart: A Week-by-Week Guide to Development (2019).*

Between week three and four, your baby will start doing two interesting things. He/she will want to snuggle closer to you, which is one of the best feelings in the world. You'll also notice other sounds than crying. It will be a gurgle or a coo, however. Don't expect them to start reciting Shakespeare until they're at least 16. And even then it's a long shot.

By week six you'll receive the first real smile. You may notice them smiling earlier than that, but that's nothing more than the relief from a wind that's been stuck for a while. This smile will mean something, as it will be directed at you.

By week 10 the baby will be able to notice your face in a crowd. In the following weeks he/she will also be more aware of their surroundings. This includes a fascination with their hands, which he/she will stare at for ages.

At week 19 the baby should have the ability to form both consonants and vowels. It's still a while before the first word, but you can help them along by pointing to things and telling them what the name for it is.

Week 22 is an interesting one, because that's when a baby starts putting everything around them in their mouth. Before this happens, you might want to give the house a thorough sweep to ensure there's nothing hazardous within reach.

By week 30 the days of finding the baby where you left them are over. He/she will become mobile. Some babies crawl quite early on, while others do a sort of army crawl on their stomach. By week 38, they'll start exploring the idea of cause and effect. This will result in a messy house, as they'll turn over just about anything that isn't nailed down.

At week 45 you'll experience the first sign of independence. The baby might start grabbing the spoon from you to feed themselves. He/she has been watching you at the dinner table for a while now, and they learn from example. Let them try it out, but be aware that it's going to be a messy affair, as almost nothing will end up in their mouths. I do have some advice for this phase, however. Use a second spoon. While they dig in and chuck their food all over the place, you can keep on feeding with the second spoon.

Soon you'll arrive at week 50, and you'll notice there's not much baby left. They're far more aware of the world around them, and they're fascinated by it. It's perfectly fine during the day, but less so at night. You might want to go to bed, but the baby is suffering from FOMO (or, Fear Of Missing Out). This is when you need to establish a strict nighttime routine, so he/she knows that it's time to go to sleep.

Before you know it, it's week 52. Your baby is exactly one year old. This is the most likely point at which he/she will first start saying 'mama' or 'papa.'

You can also give yourself a pat on the back, because you managed one of the toughest endeavors out there: you kept a baby alive for a full year.

That's why I'm all for having alcoholic beverages at a child's first birthday party. Some may think it's inappropriate, but if ever there was an occasion to celebrate with a beer, this is it.

Judging Other Parents

Raising a child is hard work, and there are many different ways to go about it. Which is why you should never judge the choices other parents make. Sure, you can gossip in private with your wife, but don't ever express your concerns to somebody's face, or in a group setting.

The only time judging another parent is acceptable is when their kids are standing on the rear seat of a car, instead of being strapped down. This makes me absolutely furious, and I usually honk to get their attention. If we happened to stop next to each other at the robot, I'll tell the parent their child should be strapped down, like some self-righteous safety belt police. More often than not, I get the finger. I don't care, however. Not strapping your kids down borders on child abuse. If you need proof, watch some safety crash tests on *YouTube*…

During my time spent with other parents, I've noticed that people tend to have extremely strong opinions on three things: breastfeeding, spanking and gender identity.

As a man, I feel as if I shouldn't even have a say in breastfeeding, but I do have some experience on the topic. Like I said before in this book, my wife was unable to breastfeed, but we have close friends that had a baby boy three months after our son was born.

The first time they came over for a visit, she asked if it was okay to breastfeed while we were chatting. My wife told her to go ahead and do it. So there I was, in a room with another woman that I've known since university. I've never seen her naked, nor have I ever wanted to. And she proceeds to just whip out a breast.

Was it strange? No, not even slightly. It's all about context, and to me that breast was nothing more than a feeding device. No sexier than the bottles on our kitchen counter.

I know it's a controversial issue, because for some weird reason female nipples are considered obscene. To me it really just boils down to the occasion. There are moments when I enjoy breasts very much, but that's in a completely different setting. When they're used for feeding, they're as asexual to me as my phone.

The second controversial topic is spanking. To most people this is a black and white topic, and they'll fiercely express their opinions both for and against. I've heard them all. "My parents spanked me and I turned out just fine," or "spanking is cruel, and should be considering child abuse."

Science isn't much help either. Do some extra reading on the topic and you'll see that there are decent, well-researched studies on both. So, what's my opinion?

Honestly, I'm apathetic about it. I don't spank my kids, because it doesn't work on them. Spanking just isn't the right punishment for either of them. If it were, I'd have no problem using it as a method.

The final topic that gets people hot under the collar is gender identity. With this I have loads of experience. My oldest is extremely flamboyant, loves to dance, loves pink, and has an impressive collection of *Barbies*.

It started when he was around five years old, and I was teaching him the value of money. He saved up some money that he received for his birthday, and for doing some chores around the house. One day he asked if he could go to the toy store, and he headed straight for the *Barbie* section. He chose one, and said that it's what he wanted.

To me this was a defining moment. I could tell him to put it back, because it wasn't appropriate, or I could let him have it. I let him have it, because I'm a firm believer of gender equality, and I want to instill those same beliefs in my sons. Had I told him he couldn't have it, it would have been the first lesson on the inferiority of women. I mean, if we can't play with girls' toys, there must be something wrong with them?

For months we'd get sideways glances from other people when we were in the shops and *Barbie* was along for the ride. I only lost my cool once when a grown man my age made fun of my son. Much to the dismay of my wife, I decided to confront this man. I asked him how fragile his masculinity must be, if he deemed it appropriate to make fun of a five-year-old.

Here's the truth fellas: It doesn't matter if your son wants to play with a *Barbie*. The most likely reason is that he just likes it. There's nothing to worry about. Children only start to form some basic sense of sexuality at six years old, and even then they're not even thinking about relationships.

Chapter 12: Raising Kids in the Modern World

My son is six years old and he already has an e-mail address.

Not one he created for himself, but rather one that was given to him by his school. He'll keep it until he's old enough to communicate directly with the school, but for now it's just a way for the school to keep in touch with parents.

Neither of them understands the concept of advertising on the television. I never allowed them to watch YouTube, until this famous video website set up an app specifically aimed at kids. Before that it was only Netflix, which has a dedicated children's platform with age appropriate content.

Obviously, I wanted to spend the first few days watching it with them, just to make sure the content on YouTube kids is safe. I applaud the company for creating this app, but with literally millions of videos going up each day, it's impossible to filter everything.

After watching the first video, an ad popped up. At the age of six and three, this was the very first time either of them had encountered such a thing.

"Why is it doing that?" they asked.

"Oh, that's just an ad. It will go away in a few seconds," I said.

"Can't you make it go away now?" they asked.

I told them back when I was young, you couldn't just decide what you wanted to watch when you wanted to watch it. And you had to sit through the commercials, because, well, that's just what we did.

Because of my background in technology, I'm constantly thinking about the world they'll grow up in. Advancement is part of life, but there are certain parts of it that keeps me awake at night.

My oldest already wants his own YouTube channel. He's a big fan of Ryan's Toys Review, and other YouTube channels like it. He wants to share his life, and his toys with the whole world, but he can't understand why I won't allow him to do that. I found a rather nice compromise, however. I regularly film him doing his crafts, and I then edit these videos on my phone to make them a bit more interesting. They never go live anywhere online, but at least he gets to see videos of himself presenting.

At least he's still a few years away from getting his own social media profiles, but we'll delve into that shortly.

First, I want to address what you should and shouldn't share on your own social media profile. As a media practitioner, part of my job was studying social media in detail, and I can tell you right off the bat that there are many reasons you shouldn't post images of your kids on social media.

There's identity theft, and naturally the danger that some sort of dodgy character could easily track your every move.

Yet, I have social media, and I regularly post images of my kids on there. There are two ways to ensure your kids' safety, and both are easy to implement. First, ensure that your phone's location services are turned off at all times. Not just for the safety of your kids, but for your own safety as well. Secondly, ensure that your privacy settings on social media are set to the most extreme setting.

Why do I do it? Well, my siblings are scattered across the globe. With all of us scattered across multiple time zones, it's the easiest way to see what everyone is up to.

Having said that, there's no getting away from social media's smart algorithms. Facebook is very much aware that I have two boys, and the moment any sort of holiday where presents are involved comes around, it will start showing me all sorts of gift ideas.

Invasion of Privacy

Do small kids have any right to privacy?

Yes, I think so. At least at home. My oldest always used the bathroom with the door open, but more recently he prefers the door closed. I respect that. He's obviously starting to set his own boundaries, which I have to respect.

Outside the confines of my house is a different story. He has a smartwatch with a GPS tracking device, and I've set up a geofence where he's allowed to move when he goes out of the house without direct supervision from us. At the moment, it's just school. There's a part of me that feels guilty about it, but I told him exactly what it was and what it did, and he's more than happy to wear it.

At some point, he won't be, and I'll be fine to take it back. If I raise him properly, he'll be able to judge whether a situation is dangerous.

Privacy is a difficult juggling act. From my side I'm simply trying to keep one of the most precious things in my life safe, but I can't do it at the expense of his own privacy.

It's easy when they're small, but it gets much harder as they get older and grow more independent.

One of the things that come with independence is a phone.

When to Buy Them a Phone

To be honest, I didn't think this particular question would cross my path as quickly as it did. But, one day, not long after starting school, my son arrived at home asking when we were going to buy him a phone. According to him, there were at least six kids in his 30-strong classroom who had phones...

These phones obviously caused havoc, because not long after we received a message from the school asking us not to send the kids to school with phones. I know exactly why. Those first few days of school are hard. It's the greatest number of hours a child has ever gone without a parent or a loved one. My son would get in the car after school every day and complain about how long it felt. The kids with phones obviously had a means to contact home and explain that they had had enough now, thank you very much.

I've thought about this for a long time, and I think the right age is around 13. At that age they'll have a bunch of friends they'll want to communicate with 24 hours a day.

But by giving them a phone, you're also granting them access to social media, and the entire world wide web.

How do you control it?

I don't think you can, but you can lay the groundwork for a healthy relationship between your child and the internet.

First and foremost, you need to warn them to take the same basic precautions to keep stalkers at bay. And then you need to warn them that what you see on social media is not an authentic representation of real life. In real life people have flaws. They don't spend their days on exotic beaches, in expensive hotels, or driving supercars. Most importantly, social media comes with all kinds of filters. Nobody actually looks that good. This is especially relevant if you have a daughter, as so many young girls develop body image problems from a young age, and the culprit is social media.

As for boys, let's get real for a moment. You're a man, I'm a man, so let's be honest. If you hand a 13-year old boy a phone, what's the first thing he's going to Google?

Yup, it's going to be boobs. It just is.

I don't necessarily know if that's a bad thing. When I was younger, adults were extremely uncomfortable when it came to anything to do with sex. Your parents would have an exceedingly excruciating talk with you, and that would be it. The rest you'd sort of have to figure out on your own.

The trick, I reckon is to find a sort of middle ground. First, you need to have an open relationship with your son. The kind of relationship where nothing is taboo, and he has the freedom to come with you with any kind of question. It's also imperative that you make him aware that pornography is also not representative of actual sexual activity, and you have to keep an eye out for any kind of porn addiction.

I know there are ways of linking phones so you can keep tabs on what your kids are watching, but this feels like a massive invasion of privacy. If anything, this will do more damage than just letting them use a device, and hope they do so responsibly.

Raising a Gentleman

My mom used to say to me, "if you want to be a man, be a gentleman."

Those words have never been more important than right now. Since the #MeToo movement, men have become more aware of the dangers women face every day. I have to admit that I was utterly clueless, which I'm ashamed about. After the bomb went off, I had a discussion with my wife, and just listening to the kind of stuff she has the deal with on a daily basis makes my blood boil.

As fathers, we have a responsibility to raise a new generation of men. We can get rid of toxic masculinity, bad behavior, rape culture, gender-based violence, all in one generation.

The secret is respect and tolerance. From a young age, you need to explain to your son that everyone is equal, and should be treated as such. No means no, and wearing pink and crying doesn't make you any less of a man.

I'm definitely not talking about taking the man out of them completely. I think some things are just hardwired into us from a young age. My two boys couldn't be more different, yet they have certain inherent characteristics. They like to play rough, get muddy, and they're particularly fond of finding new and creative ways to injure themselves.

Getting rid of toxic masculinity does not mean getting rid of masculinity completely. It's the first word that's the problem, the second one less so. There's nothing wrong with being a man, you just have to be a decent man.

I'll give you a good example of how we tried and failed at modern, woke parenting. My wife and I are fiercely anti-gun. I respect anyone's right to own one, but it's not for me. Obviously, it's a lesson I wanted to teach my own sons, so we had this stupid (in hindsight) rule that no toy guns would be allowed in the house.

So, imagine my surprise when I heard them playing outside making shooting noises. Turns out they found some sticks that sort of looked like guns and they were pretend shooting at each other.

It's then I realized that the fight against toxic masculinity wasn't a fight against all masculinity. There are just certain parts that we need to remove, and it can all be done by just setting a good example.

As the man in their life, you are the gold standard for what they will eventually become. And as I said before, if you have a daughter, you will be the gold standard for how she will want to be treated by another man in the future.

Teaching them equality is obvious, so I won't delve into that.

There are, however, two things you can do to set a good example. The number one thing is to show them that it's okay to express emotion. It's fine to be sad sometimes, and it's okay to be angry. Show them how to express those emotions in a healthy way. Some people might not agree, stating that we're raising a generation of men that simply aren't resilient enough. I don't think the two are mutually exclusive. In fact, I think they complement each other nicely.

Expressing emotion doesn't lead to a decline in resilience. I actually think it's the opposite. If one is open and honest about emotions, and you know how to cope with them thanks to a strong father figure, will that not make you more resilient to the dumpster fire that is adulting? I think so.

My second tip is to just be kind. Whether it's greeting somebody in the park, or giving a homeless person a few bucks, it teaches kids the same thing. All humans are worthy of kindness.

Chapter 13: Life Hacks

Over the years I've picked up a number of life hacks when it comes to kids, and I thought it would be nice to share them here. Most of them I only discovered with my second child, so I hope by imparting this knowledge to you now, it will actually mean something when your first child arrives.

My first hack is to get a new phone with a nice camera. I didn't know it back then, but I would eventually take thousands of photos of my offspring. Problem was, I was doing it with a smartphone with a cracked camera lens. All the images I have of him now are hazy at best, almost as if some sort of ghost snuck into each and every photo. I promise you this: You will want to document everything he/she does, no matter how mundane. So, invest in a smartphone with a good camera.

My second life hack extends to life in general. Life is too short for bad coffee, and you'll be needing a lot of it to keep you awake during those long nights. Yes, instant does the job, but you're going to have enough problems as it is. Don't add bad coffee to that list.

Along the same lines, invest in a one pan/pot cookbook. Learn how to make easy food for you and your wife. There are loads of recipe books out there aimed at making fast, healthy food without using half the utensils in the kitchen. Once the baby goes to bed, you'll want to get to bed as soon as possible. Imagine having to clean a messy kitchen before you get to climb in between the sheets...

Calming a crying baby does strange things to a person. Listing all the things I tried would eventually end up being a book all by itself. There was one method that seemed to be universally applicable. It worked on both my sons, and both my nieces. It sounds strange, but give them a tour of the house. I used to walk all over the house, telling my sons, "this is where we eat, this is where we bathe, this is where we sleep," and so on. I have no idea why it worked, but it did. And then there's the tried and trusted method of putting the child in a car and driving around until they sleep.

This brings me neatly to my next life hack. Never say never. I've heard it so many times before. "I'll never be one of those parents that drive around at 2 a.m. at night, waiting for the baby to fall asleep." Sure, buddy. Just wait until you get there. There were points where I would have driven from New York to L.A. just to get the baby to sleep.

Finally, I'd urge you to embrace the #dadlife. Make peace with the fact that you'll never be cool again, and own it. As a dad, you are now entitled to make silly puns, and nobody can judge you for it. Being a dad is also a great opportunity to make new friends. I initially kicked hard against this concept, but eventually agreed to go to various picnics and dinner parties with new people. My wife, being semi-extroverted, was happy to meet new people. My argument was that I didn't need new friends, and why should I hang with people I have nothing in common with, except that we have kids?

The thing is, it's great to hang out with these people. They don't get angry when you leave a party early when a child isn't feeling too well. They don't get upset when you tell them you won't be attending an event because you're just too tired. They get it in a way your friends without kids just don't. These friends are also a useful source of information. You can give each other tips, and they won't get offended when you refer to your own three-year-old using colorful language. In case you're wondering, it's perfectly fine to call your own child a dirty word (begins with an 'a,' ends with 'hole') behind their back. Every other person with kids will get it, I promise you.

On to more serious things. Teach your kids water safety as soon as you can. There are too many stories of babies and toddlers drowning, and it can be so easily avoided. Kids should be taught to be water-smart as soon as possible. You may have a fence around your pool at home, but you don't have complete control of the world around you. Trust me, investing in swimming classes is one of the best decisions you'll ever make.

There will also come a time when your child prefers the mother over you. Don't worry, or feel offended by it. It's just a phase they go through. My first son did it with his mom, while our second child did it to me. I eventually started referring to him as my clam, because he wouldn't budge from my hip.

The final serious life hack has to do with being the fun parent. As dads, I think we're hardwired to see our kids as fun, while mothers see them as a responsibility. I struggled for ages to act as a disciplinarian, but I had to do it. Being the fun one is unfair to the other parent, no matter how much you enjoy it.

The fact is, they have to be the bad guy all the time, and that takes a toll. There shouldn't be a fun parent and a strict parent. There should be mutual parenting, with both parents enforcing the rule, and, more importantly, getting to partake in the joys of parenthood.

Having said that, I'm still a sucker sometimes. When mom is enjoying an afternoon nap, I'll often buy the three of us an ice cream, even though sugary stuff isn't allowed after a certain amount of time. Just be cautious. A six-year-old knows when to keep his mouth shut, but a three-year-old will bust you without thinking twice.

Talking to Other Dads

I was reading a biography recently, and in it the author describes her father as being a lovely, but haunted man. He seemed to be stuck in an infinite loop with his family, going through the motions. One night he snapped, and tried to set the living room on fire. He also tried suicide a few times, and eventually settled on alcohol to numb whatever it was that was bothering him.

All of this happened in the 60s, back when men were men, and they didn't talk about their feelings. I wish I could say that things have changed, but they haven't. Not really.

The American Foundation for Suicide Prevention provides a Suicide Report (Anonymous, 2018) on their website. Men are nearly four times more likely to die from suicide than women, and middle-aged men have the highest rate of suicide. I expect these figures to rise this year, given that so many men lost their jobs, leaving them without a means of looking after their family.

I'm very lucky in the sense that I don't suffer from depression, but I am highly susceptible to anxiety.

We need to get over the idea that admitting weakness somehow makes you less of a man. In fact, in the modern world, I can't think of anything more courageous than coming out and saying, "listen, guys, I'm not doing okay."

You'd be surprised at the positive response you receive. I know this, because I've done the research. While writing this book, I asked a few of my closest friends if they'd be open to discussing their own journey to fatherhood, and it's always the same consistent fears that came up.

Because of these discussions I'm guessing I became the go-to guy for guys who just needed to vent. During the strictest lockdown phases of 2020, I received numerous phone calls from my male friends. They wouldn't come out and say that they were feeling depressed, down or anxious, but when somebody calls you "just to chat," you sort of know something's not right.

I guess if something good came out of the COVID-19 crisis, it's the fact that people aren't as ashamed of having bad things happen to them as before. Millions of people lost their jobs. I don't have a single friend who wasn't impacted by this virus in some way, shape or form.

It's nothing to be ashamed of anymore, and I'm experiencing more men being open about their mental state. Previously you'd ask how things were going and you'd get the standard, "nothing to complain about." Now people are more honest, and they'll tell you if they're not feeling okay.

Think about this within the context of raising a child, especially a son. As a young man I was taught to bottle up my feelings, which is probably the reason I'm such an anxious person today. Hopefully, my sons will see that it's okay for two men to share their feelings with each other.

It sets a great example, and I hope that it eventually leads to a drop in the suicide rate when their generation gets on with the business of adulting.

Conclusion

Why did you choose this book? The most likely answer is that you want to be a great dad. I'll let you in on a secret: you already are. You're invested in it enough to read an entire book about it, and I'm willing to bet this isn't the only one you will be reading.

The aim of this book was to simply share my experiences as a father. It has been an epic ride, and by far the most rewarding experience of my life. I love both of them to bits, even now as they're trying to beat down my office door to get my attention.

I can summarize this book in two easy to remember words: be present. At the end of the day, their most basic need is just for you to be there when you need them.

But just in case you're looking for something more prolific, here's some additional advice on how to be a great dad.

How To Be A Great Dad

I never wanted this book to feel preachy, though this last part might feel a little like that. Rest assured, these are just some thoughts I've had over the years. Your path to being a great dad might look different.

Spend Real Time With Them

I was listening to an interview with Howard Stern a few years ago, and he revealed why he got into radio. He would take rides with his dad, but instead of talking to his kids, he would turn up the radio. Stern said he decided then that he'd get a job in radio, if only to get his dad's attention.

This bit of personal information struck me hard, and made me realize that there is a difference between spending time with your kids, and spending real time with your kids. I realized I was also guilty of spending time with them, but not being present in the moment. While they were playing outside, I'd often sit in the garden reading a book. To me this counted as spending time with my kids, but in hindsight it just wasn't.

These days I give them my full attention whenever we're together. It's tougher than it sounds, because in the modern world there are so many distractions. During our playtime, I leave my phone in the house. If there's a real emergency, somebody can phone my wife, or the home phone. As a dad, you need to set strict boundaries when it comes to work time and personal time.

A child psychologist friend of mine told me something profound a few years ago. As mentioned earlier in this book, most kids don't remember anything that happened in the first three years of their life, but they do remember emotions.

Whatever you do with your child is of little significance. It doesn't need to be an expensive trip to the movies. It can be something as simple as wrestling in the garden. They won't remember what you did, but they'll always associate you with the elation they felt whenever you spent time together.

Be A Role Model

Children learn by example. This should always be at the back of your mind when raising kids.

We live in troubled times, and I firmly believe that we have an opportunity to fix all these problems by setting a good example for our kids. In a world marred by poverty, inequality, racism, and an inability to understand, you as a dad can make a real difference.

One example of this is simply loving your wife. As the father of two sons, I'm always aware of how I treat their mother. Once they're older, I'll tell them that women experience the world a lot different than we do as men.

I've also banned any form of racist talk in my house. It simply isn't allowed, and if you don't follow the rules, I have no problems asking you to leave.

At some point they will start asking difficult questions. The COVID-19 pandemic had a devastating effect on the whole world, so each night my wife would add an extra sentence into the night prayers, asking God to look after the homeless.

My eldest had some questions about the homeless after that. These kinds of questions should be approached with caution, because you always want to tell a child more than he needs to know. A part of me wanted to explain the entire pandemic, and how it cost millions of people their income. But we eventually settled on telling him that some people aren't as lucky as we are, which is why we should appreciate the things we have even more.

Finally, teach them to communicate properly. As someone with a degree in communications, I've picked up an alarming phenomenon over the last few years. Nobody listens to understand anymore. It seems like the whole world is simply listening, only to respond and voice their own opinion.

The world needs more empathy, and the only way to achieve that is by listening. I reckon half the tension in the world could be relieved if people simply took a moment to actively listen to someone else's problems. We have way more in common than we think. We may disagree on politics, global warming, whether the earth is flat or not, and gun control, but at our core we all want the same things. We want to be loved, heard, and respected.

Give The Finger To Tradition

I'm often complimented for being a good father, because I take the kids to school, spend alone time with them, change their diapers, give them a bath, and put them to bed at night. In addition to that, I also help out around the house. I wash the dishes, mop the floors, make the beds in the morning, and cook dinner every other night.

Most of the compliments come from my wife's friends, and it might surprise you that these compliments anger me. I'm also angered whenever my mom finds out I'll be looking after the kids for the evening, whenever my wife goes out with her mom or friends. She always says she's willing to come over and help me out.

I don't like these compliments, because it implies that it's not the standard way of living. When I married my wife, I agreed to be her partner. I also see her as my equal in every way, so why on earth wouldn't I help out around the house?

My wife has this fantastic book, dating back to the 1950s. I won't name the author here, because I'm not in the habit of making fun of someone else's hard work. It's a complete guide to etiquette for women, and we love reading passages out of it for fun.

According to this book, my wife is supposed to wait for me at the door, slippers in hand. The kids should already be clean, and dinner should be prepared. We're only allowed to eat, once I've had time to sit in front of the fire and read the day's newspaper. If only.

These stereotypical gender roles should be put out to pasture. The days of a woman waiting at the door with slippers are long gone, and if you still live in that world you should be ashamed.

The same goes for my kids. I know of quite a few dads who refuse to change diapers. That simply wouldn't work in my house. The kids are just as much my responsibility as they are my wife's, and that's how it works.

I don't need help babysitting my own kids. In fact, I despise the word 'babysitting.' In my world it's called parenting, and I'm just as well equipped to do it as my wife. I don't need any help looking after my own kids, mom.

This ties in nicely with setting a good example. The only thanks I want is from my sons' future wives (or husbands) for setting a high standard, and for raising two young men that treat them with respect.

Go Forth And Prosper

I hope this book put your mind at ease about having kids.

Sure, there are days I want to pull my own hair out, but those days are few and far between. On most days, I consider myself blessed. I wouldn't change a single thing about my kids, though I do sometimes wish they came with a mute button.

I'm six years into this journey, and I still have a long way to go. There are so many milestones that are still left. Soon my oldest will be going to school, where I'm fairly sure he'll hear about a few things that I'll need to explain afterwards.

Soon after that, we'll enter the teenage years. I'll be deeply uncool for a few years, but I sincerely hope that they feel safe enough to always come to me with any problems they experience.

My wife does make a good point about the teenage years, however. When they get angry with me now, they go sit in their rooms. Unfortunately, I still have to check on them every now and again, because they still need to be fed. Teenagers can make their own sandwiches, so if they do get angry with me, I'll at least get a few hours of silence.

After that they'll go to college, and I'll lay awake at night wondering if they're safe.

And soon after that they'll marry, have their own kids and then, finally, I'll be cool again. I'll be the number one source of advice, because I've been through it all. Hopefully I do a good enough job that I'm the default source. Perhaps that's the final affirmation that I did a good enough job?

What I can tell you is that it goes by so quickly. On the nights you feel desperately tired, and the baby is trying his best to burst your eardrums, it might not feel that way. But then you wake up one morning, it's six years later, and he doesn't need your help to turn on the television anymore.

That's the final thought I'll leave you with: Enjoy being a dad, because it goes by fast.

References

Arshi. (2019, June 25). Baby Facts: These 25 Amazing Facts About Babies Will Surprise You. MomJunction. https://www.momjunction.com/articles/truly-amazing-facts-about-babies_00389141/

Asmundsson, L. (2019, November 3). Baby Milestones Chart: A Week-by-Week Guide to Development. Parents.Com. https://www.parents.com/baby/development/growth/baby-development-week-by-week/

National Fatherhood Initiative. (2019). Father Absence Statistics. www.Fatherhood.Org; National Fatherhood Initiative. https://www.fatherhood.org/father-absence-statistic#:~:text=According%20to%20the%20U.S.%20Census

Nierenberg, C. (2017, December 22). Mood Swings & Mommy Brain: The Emotional Challenges of Pregnancy. Livescience.Com; Live Science. https://www.livescience.com/51043-pregnancy-emotions.html

CPSIA information can be obtained
at www.ICGtesting.com
Printed in the USA
LVHW051111241120
672558LV00004B/409